# Otolaryngology

*Editor*

C. MATTHEW STEWART

# MEDICAL CLINICS
# OF NORTH AMERICA

www.medical.theclinics.com

*Consulting Editor*
BIMAL H. ASHAR

November 2018 • Volume 102 • Number 6

# ELSEVIER

1600 John F. Kennedy Boulevard • Suite 1800 • Philadelphia, Pennsylvania, 19103-2899

http://www.theclinics.com

MEDICAL CLINICS OF NORTH AMERICA Volume 102, Number 6
November 2018 ISSN 0025-7125, ISBN-13: 978-0-323-64129-6

Editor: Jessica McCool
Developmental Editor: Kristen Helm

Medical Clinics of North America (ISSN 0025-7125) is published bimonthly by Elsevier Inc., 360 Park Avenue South, New York, NY 10010-1710. Months of publication are January, March, May, July, September, and November. Business and editorial offices: 1600 John F. Kennedy Boulevard, Suite 1800, Philadelphia, PA 19103-2899. Periodicals postage paid at New York, NY, and additional mailing offices. Subscription prices are USD $273.00 per year (US individuals), $574.00 per year (US institutions), $100.00 per year (US Students), $336.00 per year (Canadian individuals), $746.00 per year (Canadian institutions), $200.00 per year (Canadian and foreign students), $402.00 per year (foreign individuals), and $746.00 per year (foreign institutions). To receive student/resident rate, orders must be accompanied by name of affiliated institution, date of term, and the signature of program/residency coordinator on institution letterhead. Orders will be billed at individual rate until proof of status is received. Foreign air speed delivery is included in all Clinics' subscription prices. All prices are subject to change without notice. **POSTMASTER:** Send address changes to *Medical Clinics of North America*, Elsevier Health Sciences Division, Subscription Customer Service, 3251 Riverport Lane, Maryland Heights, MO 63043. **Customer Service: Telephone: 1-800-654-2452** (U.S. and Canada); **1-314-447-8871** (outside U.S. and Canada). **Fax: 314-447-8029.** E-mail: **journalscustomerserviceusa@elsevier.com** (for print support); **journalsonlinesupport-usa@elsevier.com** (for online support).

*Reprints.* For copies of 100 or more of articles in this publication, please contact the Commercial Reprints Department, Elsevier Inc., 360 Park Avenue South, New York, NY 10010-1710. Tel.: 212-633-3874; Fax: 212-633-3820; E-mail: reprints@elsevier.com.

*Medical Clinics of North America* is also published in Spanish by McGraw-Hill Interamericana Editores S. A., P.O. Box 5-237, 06500 Mexico, D.F., Mexico.

*Medical Clinics of North America* is covered in *MEDLINE/PubMed (Index Medicus), Current Contents, ASCA, Excerpta Medica, Science Citation Index,* and *ISI/BIOMED.*

## PROGRAM OBJECTIVE
The goal of the *Medical Clinics of North America* is to keep practicing physicians up to date with current clinical practice by providing timely articles reviewing the state of the art in patient care.

## TARGET AUDIENCE
All practicing physicians and other healthcare professionals.

## LEARNING OBJECTIVES
Upon completion of this activity, participants will be able to:
1. Review diagnostic testing and treatment approaches for common rhinologic conditions, chronic ear disease, and tinnitus.
2. Discuss speech and swallow rehabilitation treatment options.
3. Recognize manifestations of systemic disease and urgent infection of the head and neck.

## ACCREDITATION
The Elsevier Office of Continuing Medical Education (EOCME) is accredited by the Accreditation Council for Continuing Medical Education (ACCME) to provide continuing medical education for physicians.

The EOCME designates this enduring material for a maximum of 15 *AMA PRA Category 1 Credit*(s)™. Physicians should claim only the credit commensurate with the extent of their participation in the activity.

All other healthcare professionals requesting continuing education credit for this enduring material will be issued a certificate of participation.

## DISCLOSURE OF CONFLICTS OF INTEREST
The EOCME assesses conflict of interest with its instructors, faculty, planners, and other individuals who are in a position to control the content of CME activities. All relevant conflicts of interest that are identified are thoroughly vetted by EOCME for fair balance, scientific objectivity, and patient care recommendations. EOCME is committed to providing its learners with CME activities that promote improvements or quality in healthcare and not a specific proprietary business or a commercial interest.

**The planning committee, staff, authors and editors listed below have identified no financial relationships or relationships to products or devices they or their spouse/life partner have with commercial interest related to the content of this CME activity:**
Nishant Agrawal, MD; Yuri Agrawal, MD, MPH; Lee M. Akst, MD; Bimal H. Ashar, MD, MBA, FACP; Kofi Boahene, MD; Divya A. Chari, MD; Monika Chmielewska, DO; Vaninder K. Dhillon, MD; Susan D. Emmett, MD, MPH; Zhen Gooi, MD; David Kaylie, MD; Alison Kemp; Paige M. Kennedy, MD; John Kokesh, MD; Charles J. Limb, MD; Nyall R. London Jr, MD, PhD; Tiffany Lyon, MS, CCC-SLP; Jessica McCool; Johnathan D. McGinn, MD, FACS; Sara Mixter, MD, MPH; Annie E. Moroco, BS; Carrie L. Nieman, MD, MPH; James A. Owusu, MD; Kristine Pietsch, MA, CCC-SLP; Murugappan Ramanathan Jr, MD, FACS; Marika D. Russell, MD, FACS; Matthew S. Russell, MD, FACS; Michael C. Schubert, PT, PhD; Anil R. Shah, MD; Sharmeen Sorathia; Rosalyn W. Stewart, MD, MBA, MS; C. Matthew Stewart, MD, PhD, FACS; Sandra Stinnett, MD; Jeyanthi Surendrakumar; Kenneth Yan, MD, PhD.

**The planning committee, staff, authors and editors listed below have identified financial relationships or relationships to products or devices they or their spouse/life partner have with commercial interest related to the content of this CME activity:**
**Frank R. Lin, MD, PhD:** is a consultant/advisor for Boehringer Ingelheim International GmbH, Amplifon Hearing Health Care, and Cochlear Ltd.
**Nicholas S. Reed, AuD:** is a consultant/advisor to Clearwater Clinical.

## UNAPPROVED/OFF-LABEL USE DISCLOSURE
The EOCME requires CME faculty to disclose to the participants:
1. When products or procedures being discussed are off-label, unlabelled, experimental, and/or investigational (not US Food and Drug Administration [FDA] approved); and
2. Any limitations on the information presented, such as data that are preliminary or that represent ongoing research, interim analyses, and/or unsupported opinions. Faculty may discuss information about pharmaceutical agents that is outside of FDA-approved labelling. This information is intended solely for CME and is not intended to promote off-label use of these medications. If you have any questions, contact the medical affairs department of the manufacturer for the most recent prescribing information.

## TO ENROLL

To enroll in the *Medical Clinics of North America* Continuing Medical Education program, call customer service at 1-800-654-2452 or sign up online at http://www.theclinics.com/home/cme. The CME program is available to subscribers for an additional annual fee of USD $300.90.

## METHOD OF PARTICIPATION

In order to claim credit, participants must complete the following:
1. Complete enrolment as indicated above.
2. Read the activity.
3. Complete the CME Test and Evaluation. Participants must achieve a score of 70% on the test. All CME Tests and Evaluations must be completed online.

## CME INQUIRIES/SPECIAL NEEDS

For all CME inquiries or special needs, please contact elsevierCME@elsevier.com.

# MEDICAL CLINICS OF NORTH AMERICA

---

**ISSUE OF RELATED INTEREST**

*Physician Assistant Clinics*, April 2018 (Vol. 3, No. 2)
**Otolaryngology**
Laura A. Kirk, *Editor*
Available at: http://www.physicianassistant.theclinics.com/

---

# Contributors

## CONSULTING EDITOR

**BIMAL H. ASHAR, MD, MBA, FACP**
Associate Professor of Medicine, Division of General Internal Medicine, Johns Hopkins School of Medicine, Baltimore, Maryland, USA

## EDITOR

**C. MATTHEW STEWART, MD, PhD, FACS**
Associate Professor, Department of Otolaryngology–Head and Neck Surgery, Johns Hopkins School of Medicine, The Johns Hopkins Hospital, Baltimore, Maryland, USA

## AUTHORS

**NISHANT AGRAWAL, MD**
Section of Otolaryngology, Department of Surgery, The University of Chicago Medicine, Chicago, Illinois, USA

**YURI AGRAWAL, MD, MPH**
Associate Professor, Department of Otolaryngology–Head and Neck Surgery, Johns Hopkins School of Medicine, Baltimore, Maryland, USA

**LEE M. AKST, MD**
Department of Otolaryngology–Head and Neck Surgery, Johns Hopkins School of Medicine, Baltimore, Maryland, USA

**KOFI BOAHENE, MD**
Department of Otorhinolaryngology–Head and Neck Surgery, The Johns Hopkins Hospital, Baltimore, Maryland, USA

**DIVYA A. CHARI, MD**
Resident Physician, Department of Otolaryngology–Head and Neck Surgery, University of California, San Francisco, San Francisco, California, USA

**MONIKA CHMIELEWSKA, DO**
ENT Associates, Grand Blanc, Michigan, USA

**VANINDER K. DHILLON, MD**
Assistant Professor, Department of Otolaryngology–Head and Neck Surgery, Johns Hopkins School of Medicine, Baltimore, Maryland, USA

**SUSAN D. EMMETT, MD, MPH**
Assistant Professor of Surgery and Global Health, Head and Neck Surgery and Communication Sciences, Duke University School of Medicine, Duke Global Health Institute, Durham, North Carolina, USA

**ZHEN GOOI, MD**
Section of Otolaryngology, Department of Surgery, The University of Chicago Medicine, Chicago, Illinois, USA

**DAVID KAYLIE, MD**
Associate Professor of Surgery, Head and Neck Surgery and Communication Sciences, Duke University School of Medicine, Durham, North Carolina, USA

**PAIGE M. KENNEDY, MD**
Department of Otolaryngology–Head and Neck Surgery, The University of Chicago Medicine, The University of Chicago Medicine and Biological Sciences, Chicago, Illinois, USA

**JOHN KOKESH, MD**
Director, Department of Otolaryngology, Alaska Native Medical Center, Anchorage, Alaska, USA

**CHARLES J. LIMB, MD**
Professor, Chief of Division of Otology, Neurotology, and Skull Base Surgery, Department of Otolaryngology–Head and Neck Surgery, University of California, San Francisco, San Francisco, California, USA

**FRANK R. LIN, MD, PhD**
Associate Professor, Departments of Otolaryngology–Head and Neck Surgery and Medicine, Johns Hopkins School of Medicine, Cochlear Center for Hearing and Public Health, Department of Epidemiology, Johns Hopkins Bloomberg School of Public Health, Baltimore, Maryland, USA

**NYALL R. LONDON Jr, MD, PhD**
Department of Otolaryngology–Head and Neck Surgery, Johns Hopkins School of Medicine, Baltimore, Maryland, USA

**TIFFANY LYON, MS, CCC-SLP**
Staff, Department of Speech and Language Pathology, University of Utah, Salt Lake City, Utah, USA

**JOHNATHAN D. McGINN, MD, FACS**
Division of Otolaryngology–Head and Neck Surgery, Associate Professor, Department of Surgery, Penn State Milton S. Hershey Medical Center, Hershey, Pennsylvania, USA

**SARA MIXTER, MD, MPH**
Assistant Professor, Department of Medicine, Division of General Internal Medicine, Johns Hopkins School of Medicine, Baltimore, Maryland, USA

**ANNIE E. MOROCO, BS**
Division of Otolaryngology–Head and Neck Surgery, Department of Surgery, Penn State Milton S. Hershey Medical Center, Hershey, Pennsylvania, USA

**CARRIE L. NIEMAN, MD, MPH**
Assistant Professor, Department of Otolaryngology–Head and Neck Surgery, Johns Hopkins School of Medicine, Cochlear Center for Hearing and Public Health, Johns Hopkins Bloomberg School of Public Health, Baltimore, Maryland, USA

**JAMES A. OWUSU, MD**
Department of Head and Neck Surgery, Mid-Atlantic Permanente Medical Group, McLean, Virginia, USA

**KRISTINE PIETSCH, MA, CCC-SLP**
Assistant, Department of Otolaryngology, The Johns Hopkins University, Baltimore, Maryland, USA

**MURUGAPPAN RAMANATHAN Jr, MD, FACS**
Department of Otolaryngology–Head and Neck Surgery, Johns Hopkins School of Medicine, Baltimore, Maryland, USA

**NICHOLAS S. REED, AuD**
Assistant Professor, Department of Otolaryngology–Head and Neck Surgery, Johns Hopkins School of Medicine, Cochlear Center for Hearing and Public Health, Johns Hopkins Bloomberg School of Public Health, Baltimore, Maryland, USA

**MARIKA D. RUSSELL, MD, FACS**
Associate Professor, Otolaryngology–Head and Neck Surgery, University of California, San Francisco, San Francisco, California, USA

**MATTHEW S. RUSSELL, MD, FACS**
Assistant Professor, Otolaryngology–Head and Neck Surgery, University of California, San Francisco, San Francisco, California, USA

**MICHAEL C. SCHUBERT, PT PhD**
Associate Professor, Departments of Otolaryngology–Head and Neck Surgery and Physical Medicine and Rehabilitation, Johns Hopkins School of Medicine, Baltimore, Maryland, USA

**ANIL R. SHAH, MD**
Department of Otolaryngology–Head and Neck Surgery, The University of Chicago Medicine, Chicago, Illinois, USA

**SHARMEEN SORATHIA**
MBBS Student, Ziauddin University College of Medicine, Karachi, Pakistan; Johns Hopkins School of Medicine, Baltimore, Maryland, USA

**C. MATTHEW STEWART, MD, PhD, FACS**
Associate Professor, Department of Otolaryngology–Head and Neck Surgery, Johns Hopkins School of Medicine, The Johns Hopkins Hospital, Baltimore, Maryland, USA

**ROSALYN W. STEWART, MD, MBA, MS**
Associate Professor, Department of Medicine, Division of General Internal Medicine, Johns Hopkins School of Medicine, Baltimore, Maryland, USA

**SANDRA STINNETT, MD**
Department of Otolaryngology–Head and Neck Surgery, University of Tennessee Health Science Center, Memphis, Tennessee, USA

**KENNETH YAN, MD, PhD**
Section of Otolaryngology, Department of Surgery, The University of Chicago Medicine, Chicago, Illinois, USA

# Contents

Chronic ear disease is composed of a spectrum of otologic disorders intrinsically tied to Eustachian tube dysfunction. Presentation can range from asymptomatic findings on physical examination to critically ill patients with intracranial complications. Internists represent the first line in diagnosis of these conditions, making awareness of the common signs and symptoms essential. With surgical management often required, partnership between internal medicine and otolaryngology is fundamental in the management of patients with chronic ear disease.

Objective and subjective tinnitus can often be differentiated based on comprehensive history, physical examination, and audiogram. Examples of objective tinnitus include vascular abnormalities, palatal myoclonus, patulous eustachian tube, and stapedial/tensor tympani muscle spasm. Subjective tinnitus is usually associated with hearing loss. Rarely, tinnitus is the result of an underlying condition. In these cases, imaging and additional testing may be indicated. Classification of the type, quality, and intensity of tinnitus is helpful in the work-up and treatment of tinnitus. Treatment modalities include cognitive behavioral therapy, tinnitus retraining therapy, sound therapy, hearing aids, cochlear implants, pharmacotherapy, and brain stimulation.

Systemic diseases commonly managed by the Internist may have presentations within the head and neck. Awareness of these manifestations, sometimes as the presenting signs or symptoms of systemic disease, may aid the Internist in diagnosis and management. The Otolaryngologist may be helpful in assisting in the evaluation of these patients and in some cases providing targeted symptomatic therapy. Some systemic processes can generate emergent airway events, and early engagement of the otolaryngologist is of value.

Infections of the head and neck are common and appropriately managed by primary care providers in most cases. However, some infections are associated with significant morbidity and require urgent recognition and management by specialty services. These include deep neck space infections originating in the oral cavity, pharynx, and salivary glands, as well as complicated otologic and sinonasal infection. This article provides a review of these conditions, including the pathophysiology, presenting features, and initial management strategy.

# Foreword
# Reflections

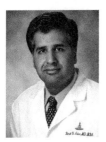

Bimal H. Ashar, MD, MBA, FACP
*Consulting Editor*

Along with the stethoscope, the head mirror has historically been one of the most recognizable devices used to depict physicians. This simple tool, consisting of a concave mirror with a small hole in the middle attached to a headband, has been a cornerstone of examination of the ear, nose, and throat. When a light source is directed at the mirror, the reflection serves to illuminate a concentrated area and enhance direct visualization. Similar to the stethoscope, its accepted use can be traced back to the 1800s. However, unlike the stethoscope, use of the head mirror is now becoming obsolete. Medical students and residents have little exposure to this time-honored device. Most primary care physicians now use the penlight for simple illumination, while most otolaryngologists have turned to the head lamp for more intricate work. Despite it becoming outdated to most, the importance of the head mirror cannot be overstated. Direct visualization of the structures of the head and neck is vital, given the prevalence of disorders affecting the ears, nose, and throat.

Diseases of the sinuses alone affect more than 11% of the US adult population yearly. Tinnitus affects about 25 million Americans, whereas hearing loss afflicts twice that number. A National Health Interview Survey found that 21% of adults had difficulty following a conversation amid background noise.[1] This number has the potential to rise with the use of personal audio devices. "Dizziness" continues to be one of the most challenging symptoms that primary care providers encounter. In addition to these "benign" conditions, serious infections of the head and neck can occur, producing devastating consequences (including death) unless diagnosed and treated rapidly, whereas nearly 14,000 people in the United States die of head and neck cancers yearly.

In this issue of *Medical Clinics of North America*, Dr Stewart has enlisted a broad array of experts who cover a number of areas seen routinely in general practice. In addition to assisting in developing approaches to common conditions, Dr Stewart and his colleagues also discuss advances made for ailments (eg, tinnitus and hearing

Med Clin N Am 102 (2018) xv–xvi
https://doi.org/10.1016/j.mcna.2018.08.015
0025-7125/18/© 2018 Published by Elsevier Inc.

loss), whose treatments have historically been considered futile. It is hoped this issue is worth some reflection.

Bimal H. Ashar, MD, MBA, FACP
Division of General Internal Medicine
Johns Hopkins University School of Medicine
601 North Caroline Street
#7143
Baltimore, MD 21287, USA

*E-mail address:*
Bashar1@jhmi.edu

**REFERENCE**

1. Zelaya CE, Lucas JW, Hoffman HJ. MMWR QuickStats: percentage of adults with selected hearing problems, by type of problem and age group—National Health Interview Survey, United States, 2014. MMWR Morb Mortal Wkly Rep 2015;64: 1058. Available at: https://www.cdc.gov/mmwr/preview/mmwrhtml/mm6437a8.htm.

# Preface

# Otolaryngology for the Internist

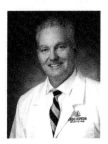

C. Matthew Stewart, MD, PhD, FACS
*Editor*

The practice of Otolaryngology involves both the medical and surgical management of disorders and diseases of the head and neck. The anatomy and function of the otolaryngology, head and neck surgeon span a wide array of cranial nerves and structures that include the special senses of olfaction, gustation, hearing, balance, and the sense of touch as well as the vital functions of breathing, chewing, swallowing, and talking. This expertise includes the nose and sinuses (rhinology); specialized care of the pediatric population; the ear, hearing, and balance (otology and neurotology); the throat, including voice and swallowing (laryngology); cosmetic, functional, and reconstructive surgery of the face (facial and plastic reconstructive surgery); benign and malignant lesions of the head and neck (head and neck oncology); and the medical and immunotherapy management of allergy.

The internist is well aware of the high incidence of new and chronic visits related to these areas of otolaryngology, head and neck surgery (more than 25 million US adults a year are diagnosed with sinusitis alone, for example). A key question for the internist is often when to escalate a chronic otolaryngology, head and surgery disorder by referral to a specialist for medical management and/or surgical intervention. In other cases, management of these disorders by the internist requires additional information and methods.

In this issue, we explore the expertise of the specialists above for a wide variety of the most common needs for the internist. These include the traditional areas above as well as an introduction to some of the most common rehabilitation areas, such as audiology, vestibular physical therapy, and speech and language pathology. These specialists play a vital role in the restoration of function in the care and management of your patients. The internist and the otolaryngologist share many patients as there are many systemic diseases that have primary or serious manifestations in the head and neck area. Internists also have an increasing population of pediatric patients with chronic health conditions that age out of pediatric practices, populating practices

Med Clin N Am 102 (2018) xvii–xviii
https://doi.org/10.1016/j.mcna.2018.08.014
0025-7125/18/© 2018 Published by Elsevier Inc.

with an increasingly complex array of disorders, including those of pediatric otolaryngology. Our authors have assembled a comprehensive review of these topics and others. We hope this issue will be of frequent use in the care and management of your patients.

C. Matthew Stewart, MD, PhD, FACS
Otolaryngology, Head and Neck Surgery
Johns Hopkins University
School of Medicine
601 North Caroline Street
JHOC Suite 6260B
Baltimore, MD, 21287, USA

*E-mail address:*
cstewa16@jhmi.edu

# Otolaryngology for the Internist: Hearing Loss

Carrie L. Nieman, MD, MPH[a,b,*], Nicholas S. Reed, AuD[a,b], Frank R. Lin, MD, PhD[a,b,c,d]

## KEYWORDS

- Hearing loss • Age-related hearing loss • Hearing health • Hearing health care
- Hearing aids • Over-the-counter hearing aids • Older adults

## KEY POINTS

- Internists can differentiate conditions presenting with hearing loss by a focused history and associated time course.
- Every patient presenting with hearing loss should undergo an otologic history and physical, including otoscopy, facial nerve examination, and tuning fork examination.
- The most urgent form of hearing loss is sudden sensorineural hearing loss, which requires audiometry and referral to an otolaryngologist, along with rapid initiation of treatment with oral steroids and/or intratympanic steroid injection.
- Age-related hearing loss is highly prevalent, and growing evidence demonstrates important implications on healthy aging. Affordable, accessible hearing care is needed, and recent national efforts, including federal legislation, are expanding options for older adults.

## INTRODUCTION

Hearing loss is the third most common chronic condition and affects more than 60 million people in the United States.[1,2] Although age-related hearing loss is the most common cause of hearing loss, there are a number of etiologies and presentations an internist must differentiate to guide appropriate treatment and referrals. This article

Disclosures: F.R. Lin is a consultant to Boehringer-Ingelheim, Amplifon, and Cochlear Ltd. N.S. Reed is a Scientific Advisory Board member for Clearwater Clinical.
[a] Department of Otolaryngology–Head and Neck Surgery, Johns Hopkins University School of Medicine, 601 North Caroline Street, Baltimore, MD 21287, USA; [b] Cochlear Center for Hearing and Public Health, Johns Hopkins Bloomberg School of Public Health, 2024 East Monument Street, Suite 2-700, Baltimore, MD 21205, USA; [c] Department of Medicine, Johns Hopkins University School of Medicine, 5200 Eastern Avenue, Baltimore, MD 21234, USA; [d] Department of Epidemiology, Johns Hopkins Bloomberg School of Public Health, 615 North Wolfe Street, Baltimore, MD 21205, USA
* Corresponding author. Department of Otolaryngology–Head and Neck Surgery, Johns Hopkins University School of Medicine, 601 North Caroline Street, JHOC 6214, Baltimore, MD 21287.
E-mail address: cnieman1@jhmi.edu

https://doi.org/10.1016/j.mcna.2018.06.013
0025-7125/18/© 2018 Elsevier Inc. All rights reserved.

reviews common acute and chronic presentations of hearing loss, and, given its prevalence, provides a primer on age-related hearing loss, including practical approaches to management.

## ACUTE HEARING LOSS
### Symptoms

Hearing loss can occur unilaterally or bilaterally and with varying severity, ranging from mild to profound loss. Depending on the severity, hearing loss can present as a sensation of aural fullness and be accompanied by symptoms such as tinnitus, vertigo, otalgia, or otorrhea. In obtaining a history, one should include details regarding onset (ie, sudden vs gradual), laterality, severity, persistence of symptoms (ie, fluctuating vs constant), and associated symptoms. Past personal and family history related to hearing and prior ear surgeries will also inform the differential diagnosis. **Box 1** provides a list of key questions when interviewing a patient over the phone or in the office.

### Diagnostic Tests

An otologic history is fundamental to differentiating common causes of acute hearing loss and should be partnered with an otologic physical examination, including otoscopy, a facial nerve examination, and a tuning fork examination. Careful examination of the pinna and otoscopy of the external auditory canal and tympanic membrane should be performed bilaterally. On placing the speculum in the ear canal, note any lesions of the ear canal. As much of the tympanic membrane as possible should be observed and the examination can be optimized by using the largest speculum possible and pulling the superior aspect of the pinna superiorly and laterally to straighten the ear canal.

Diagnostic tests related to hearing loss primarily consist of audiometry. Audiograms are typically performed by audiologists in a soundproof booth and remain the gold

---

**Box 1**
**Key questions in obtaining an otologic history**

Description of symptoms:
  Onset acute or gradual?
  Unilateral or bilateral?
  Fluctuating or constant?
  Able to use a phone on the side of the loss?

Associated symptoms:
  Vertigo?
  Tinnitus?
  Otorrhea? Color/consistency/odor associated with the fluid?
  Otalgia?

Recent history:
  Head trauma?
  Noise exposure?
  Viral illness?
  Use cotton swabs?

Past otologic history:
  Prior ear-related diagnosis?
  Prior ear surgery, including tympanostomy tubes?
  History of occupational or recreational noise exposure?

Otologic family history:
  Known family history of hearing loss or ear-related diagnoses?

standard in the diagnosis of hearing loss. Audiometry differentiates conductive from sensorineural hearing loss as well as the severity. Obtaining an audiogram can be difficult after-hours or on weekends, but mobile options are available and have been validated against traditional audiometry.[3–6] Several smartphone applications use the patient's earbuds and perform a hearing screening that tests thresholds over a range of frequencies, which can approximate hearing thresholds and inform initial management.[3–6]

## Differential Diagnosis and Associated Management

### Cerumen impaction
The hydrophobic and bacteriostatic properties of cerumen protect the external auditory canal and cerumen is eliminated from the ear canal through epithelial migration oriented laterally, making the ear canal "self-cleaning."[7,8] However, depending on individual differences in cerumen quality and quantity and use of cotton swabs, cerumen can become impacted and present with an acute or gradual change in hearing. Patients may report pruritus and aural fullness and will typically have a history of cotton swab use or other foreign objects. Patients should be counseled against using cotton swabs or any other object in the ear canal. The diagnosis is made based on physical examination, where cerumen, partially or completely, obstructs the view of the tympanic membrane. Cerumen removal through an operative otoscope or topical cerumenolytics can used be as an initial treatment. If the impaction persists, referral to an otolaryngologist for cerumen removal and microscopic examination is recommended. If the patient reports hearing improvement following cerumen removal, further diagnostic work-up, such as audiometry, is generally not warranted. Patients also can be counseled on preventive measures, including avoiding cotton swabs and routine use of emollients such as mineral oil.[9]

### Otitis externa
The primary symptoms of acute otitis externa (AOE) are otalgia, pruritus, and purulent otorrhea, but hearing loss secondary to edema of the ear canal can accompany this condition.[10] Patients present with a history of water exposure and/or manipulation of the ear canal, including cotton swabs or other foreign objects.[10] Classically, AOE presents in swimmers in the summer months, where warm, moist ear canals foster bacterial growth. Obtaining a complete history is essential, particularly related to comorbidities, namely diabetes and immune deficiencies, because these influence treatment. Physical examination findings include an erythematous and edematous ear canal, a pinna that is tender to manipulation, and purulent discharge.[10] The otorrhea and/or edema of the canal often limit the otoscopic view of the tympanic membrane. As a bacterial infection most commonly caused by *Pseudomonas aeruginosa* and *Staphylococcus aureus*, first-line treatment consists of topical antiseptic eardrops that include acetic acid and a steroid, such as hydrocortisone, or antibiotic eardrops with steroids.[11] Ciprofloxacin-based eardrops with steroids are commonly prescribed, typically twice a day for 7 to 10 days.[11] Topical treatments are most important and, to be effective, drops must be adequately delivered to the ear canal. If the patient presents with significant ear canal edema, a wick may be needed to ensure sufficient delivery of topical treatments.[11] Given the pain associated with AOE, pain control should be discussed and offered. Systemic antibiotic treatments are not the first-line treatment for AOE but may be a necessary adjunct if the patient is diabetic, has an immune deficiency, the associated edema and erythema have significantly spread beyond the ear, or topical treatments have failed to prevent progression of the disease.[11] Similar to topical treatments, systematic antibiotics should cover *P aeruginosa* and *S aureus*.

With the edema and otorrhea associated with AOE, regular debridement of the ear canal is typically needed to support recovery. A referral to an otolaryngologist should be considered if symptoms persist or progress despite initial appropriate treatment and/ or if significant debris or purulence obstructs delivery of topical eardrops and debridement and/or wick placement is needed.

Particularly severe or prolonged courses of AOE raise the possibility of malignant otitis externa, which is a complication of AOE and a potentially lethal infection that extends beyond the soft tissue of the ear canal to involve the bone of the external auditory canal and the surrounding skull base.[10,12] Generally seen in diabetic and immunocompromised patients, all cases of AOE in these patients must be treated and closely monitored for improvement.[10,12] Malignant otitis externa can be differentiated from AOE by the severity of symptoms, where severe otalgia is present for 4 or more weeks along with purulent otorrhea, and, at times, cranial neuropathies, including facial paresis or paralysis.[10,12] The defining examination finding is the presence of granulation tissue along the floor of the ear canal. Treatment requires intravenous antibiotics and optimizing management of the underlying immunosuppression and suspicion of malignant otitis externa necessitates an expedited referral to an otolaryngologist.

### Herpes zoster oticus

Hearing loss can present as a symptom of herpes zoster oticus when accompanied by otalgia and a vesicular rash in the canal.[12] When these symptoms are accompanied by facial paralysis, the condition is called Ramsay Hunt syndrome.[12] Careful examination of the ear canal to identify the classic vesicular rash of herpes zoster and the cranial nerves to identify partial or complete facial weakness are important in differentiating this condition from AOE and sudden sensorineural hearing loss. The diagnosis can be confirmed by isolating the virus from vesicular fluid.[13] Once identified, timely treatment with oral steroids (prednisone 60 mg daily for 3–5 days) and antivirals (famciclovir 500 mg 3 times a day for 7 days or acyclovir 800 mg 5 times a day for 7–10 days) are critical along with an urgent otolaryngology referral.[14,15]

### Acute otitis media

Acute otitis media can occur in adults but is much less common than in children. Among adults, otitis media often occurs in the setting of an upper respiratory tract infection or allergic rhinitis.[16] The patient presents with otalgia and decreased hearing, particularly if an effusion is present. On examination, the tympanic membrane is erythematous and often bulging with an effusion. In differentiating otitis media from otitis externa, pain with manipulation of the pinna or edema and erythema of the external auditory canal are defining symptoms of AOE but are not seen in otitis media. Treatment for uncomplicated otitis media consists of amoxicillin 500 mg three times a day for 7 to 10 days and, for patients who are diabetic or immunocompromised, treatment should consist of amoxicillin/clavulanate 875 mg twice a day or 500 mg three times a day for 10 to 14 days.[17] Referral to an otolaryngologist can allow for myringotomy performed in the office, which would provide immediate relief of the otalgia and hearing loss for the patient with evacuation of the effusion.[16] If an effusion is present for more than 8 weeks, particularly if unilateral, patients should be referred to an otolaryngologist for an examination of the nasopharynx.[18,19]

### Meniere disease

Although the predominant symptoms of Meniere disease, or endolymphatic hydrops, is episodic rotational vertigo that lasts for up to hours at a time, patients can present with fluctuating low-frequency hearing loss as well as aural fullness and tinnitus.[20,21] Symptoms are generally unilateral but symptoms can present in the contralateral ear over time. Typically, the patient's symptoms fluctuate in the beginning with recurrent attacks but eventually "burns out" and the hearing loss can become permanent.[20,21] The primary way to differentiate Meniere disease is based on the clinical history and audiometry. Patients should be referred to an otolaryngologist and seen urgently if hearing loss is sudden, as during an attack.

### Sudden sensorineural hearing loss

Among conditions that can present with an acute change in hearing, sudden sensorineural hearing loss (SSNHL) is one of the few conditions that requires emergent treatment and referral to an otolaryngologist. Patients present with unilateral hearing loss that most often occurs suddenly or over the course of 1 to 3 days.[22,23] Hearing loss can be partial or complete but is defined as at least a 30 dB hearing loss decrease in hearing thresholds across 3 frequencies.[22,23] Patients often report aural fullness and potentially a transient sense of disequilibrium or vertigo and may notice that they are not able to hear out of one ear while talking on the telephone.[22,23] SSNHL is often misdiagnosed as acute otitis media or Eustachian tube dysfunction and otitis media with effusion, which can delay care (**Table 1**). **Table 1** reviews the key history and physical examination findings to differentiate SSNHL from acute otitis media and Eustachian tube dysfunction with effusion. In addition to a tuning fork examination, mobile smartphone applications can also aid in approximating the patient's hearing when a formal audiogram may be inaccessible after-hours or on weekends. However, this preliminary hearing screening should not replace a formal audiogram but can be used to inform initial treatment. The exact mechanism of SSNHL is unknown but can be due to a viral infection, tumor, or vascular etiology. Regardless, suspected SSNHL loss requires immediate treatment. Time to treatment is an important predictor of outcome. Referral to an otolaryngologist for audiometry and further evaluation and treatment are necessary. Treatment with oral steroids (prednisone 1 mg/kg per day for 14–21 days with taper) should begin as soon as possible.[22] The otolaryngologist can also perform intratympanic steroid injections into the middle ear as an adjunct to oral steroid treatment or as a primary treatment for patients who are unable to tolerate a prolonged course of oral steroids.[22]

**Table 2** summarizes the previously described diagnoses and treatments.

## CHRONIC HEARING LOSS
### Symptoms

Hearing loss can occur gradually, over months to years, and, therefore, can be difficult for patients to have insight into their hearing status. Among the causes of hearing loss that occur gradually, hearing loss is typically progressive, beginning as a mild loss and worsening over time. The most important history to obtain is whether the hearing loss is unilateral or bilateral, where unilateral progressive hearing loss often indicates a worse underlying pathology than age-related hearing loss, which is bilateral. Patients with a gradual change in hearing can present with aural fullness. Tinnitus is also common, especially when the hearing loss has been long-standing. Vertigo and/or a sense of disequilibrium as well as otorrhea are concerning symptoms in the setting of gradual hearing loss because they point to a diagnosis other than age-related hearing loss. It is important to obtain a detailed personal and family otologic history, including a history of ear surgeries and exposure to noise, occupational and recreational, and ototoxic medications.

### Diagnostic Tests

Similar to an acute hearing loss, begin with an otologic history and physical examination, including otoscopy, a tuning fork examination, and facial nerve

**Table 1**
Differentiating sudden sensorineural hearing loss and otitis media

| | Sudden Sensorineural Hearing Loss | Acute Otitis Media | Eustachian Tube Dysfunction Otitis Media with Effusion |
|---|---|---|---|
| Main symptom | Hearing loss | Otalgia | Aural fullness |
| Secondary symptoms | Aural fullness +/− Tinnitus +/− Transient dizziness or vertigo | Aural fullness Decreased or "muffled" hearing | Decreased or "muffled hearing" |
| Degree of change in hearing | Significant change in hearing Typically *unable* to use the phone | Muffled hearing Typically able to use the phone | Muffled hearing Typically able to use the phone |
| Time course | *Sudden*, typically within minutes, always within 3 d | Over the course of days | Chronic |
| Associated history | +/− History of recent viral illness | History of recent viral illness History of allergy exacerbation | History of ear infections or prior tympanostomy tubes History of allergies |
| Otoscopic examination | *Normal* tympanic membrane Mobile tympanic membrane on pneumatic otoscopy | Erythematous tympanic membrane Bulging tympanic membrane (effusion) No mobility of tympanic membrane on pneumatic otoscopy | Bulging tympanic membrane (effusion) No mobility of tympanic membrane on pneumatic otoscopy |
| Tuning fork examination | Weber (512 or 1024 cycle) tuning fork localizes to the *contralateral* side of the involved ear | Weber (512 or 1024 cycle) tuning fork localizes to the involved (ipsilateral) side | Weber (512 or 1024 cycle) tuning fork localizes to the involved (ipsilateral) side |
| Treatment | Oral steroids Urgent referral to otolaryngologist | Oral antibiotics If uncertain, urgent referral to otolaryngologist | Nasal steroids, treat allergies If uncertain, urgent referral to otolaryngologist |

examination. In most cases, the ear examination will be normal but a thorough examination of the tympanic membrane to examine for retraction and/or keratin debris may indicate chronic otitis media and/or the presence of cholesteatoma, which requires further examination and treatment by an otolaryngologist. Obtaining an audiogram is essential and can be obtained from an audiologist or through an otolaryngologist.

### Differential Diagnosis and Associated Management

#### Chronic otitis media and cholesteatoma
Patients who present with a history of hearing loss over time and a history of ear infections as a child and/or multiple sets of tympanostomy tubes may have chronic otitis media and associated cholesteatoma.[24,25] Patients typically present with a history of purulent otorrhea as well as hearing loss, tinnitus, vertigo, and/or facial nerve palsy

**Table 2**
Common causes and initial treatments for acute hearing loss

| Causes of Acute Hearing Loss | Key History Findings | Key Physical Examination Findings | Treatment |
| --- | --- | --- | --- |
| Cerumen impaction | Gradual or acute<br>Unilateral or bilateral<br>Aural fullness<br>Pruritus<br>History of cotton swab use | Cerumen obstructing the tympanic membrane | Removal via operative otoscope<br>Cerumenolytics<br>*When to refer:* If first-line measures, unsuccessful |
| Otitis externa | Otalgia<br>Purulent otorrhea<br>History of swimming | Otalgia with manipulation of the pinna<br>Erythema, edema of canal | Topical antibiotics ± steroids<br>Wick placement<br>Frequent debridement<br>Consider oral antibiotics if immunocompromised<br>*When to refer:* If first-line measures unsuccessful; symptoms progress; more aggressive debridement or wick placement required |
| Malignant otitis externa | Severe otalgia for 4+ weeks<br>History of diabetes | Granulation tissue present in canal | Intravenous antibiotics<br>*When to refer:* Urgent immediate referral |
| Herpes zoster oticus | Otalgia<br>+/− Facial paralysis | Vesicular rash in the canal | Oral steroids<br>Oral antivirals<br>*When to refer:* Urgent immediate referral |
| Acute otitis media | Otalgia<br>History of upper respiratory infection, allergic rhinitis | Bulging, erythematous tympanic membrane | Oral antibiotics<br>*When to refer:* For immediate pain relief with office-based myringotomy<br>Unilateral effusion present for 8+ weeks |
| Meniere disease | Episodic vertigo<br>Fluctuating low-frequency hearing loss<br>Aural fullness | Nystagmus during acute attack | *When to refer:* Urgent immediate referral if hearing loss present |
| Sudden sensorineural hearing loss | Sudden hearing loss<br>Aural fullness<br>+/− Dizziness<br>History of viral illness | Normal otoscopic examination | Oral steroids<br>*When to refer:* Urgent immediate referral for audiometry, possible intratympanic steroid injection |

depending on the structures involved. On physical examination, patients may have retraction of the tympanic membrane, white skinlike debris, polypoid granulation tissue, and/or purulent fluid. For further evaluation and treatment, patients should be referred to an otolaryngologist.

### Autoimmune inner ear disease

Several systemic autoimmune diseases can also affect hearing and can mirror disease progression, leading to a progressive or fluctuating, bilateral hearing loss and can include, but are not limited to, systemic lupus erythematosus, inflammatory bowel disease, ulcerative colitis, Crohn disease, polyarteritis nodosum, and granulomatosis with polyangiitis.[26]

### Vestibular schwannoma

Patients with unilateral hearing loss without a history of trauma or prior otologic surgery may have a small benign tumor of the vestibular nerve (cranial nerve VIII). Typically, the associated hearing loss progresses slowly and affects higher frequencies. However, up to 25% of patients with vestibular schwannomas present with SSNHL.[27] Most patients also present with tinnitus, a sense of disequilibrium or vertigo, and facial paresis or paralysis. On physical examination, the tympanic membrane will appear healthy but there may be facial weakness or asymmetry, which is often subclinical. An audiogram and referral to an otolaryngologist are recommended for patients who develop unilateral hearing loss.

### Noise-induced hearing loss

Patients can present with an acute change in hearing that may be temporary or permanent following exposure to acoustic trauma, such as a brief but intense noise.[27] More frequently, patients will present with slowly progressive hearing loss and a history of prolonged noise exposure. Patients will generally have a normal otoscopic examination. Patients should have an audiogram performed and referred to an otolaryngologist. Although patients may benefit from hearing aids, prevention is critical, including minimizing exposure and routine use of hearing protective devices like earplugs.

**Table 3** summarizes the previously described diagnoses and treatments.

## AGE-RELATED HEARING LOSS
### Epidemiology

Age-related hearing loss is almost universal, in which the rates of clinically significant hearing loss almost double with each decade of life and equates to 23 million older Americans.[2,28,29] Sex and skin pigmentation are risk factors for age-related hearing loss; rates of hearing loss are higher among men versus women and among those with fairer skin color (lower Fitzpatrick skin type) versus darker skin color (higher Fitzpatrick skin type), which is believed secondary to differences in the density of protective strial melanocytes in the cochlea.[29–32] Cardiovascular risk factors, such as hypertension, diabetes, stroke, and smoking, have not been found to be significantly and consistently associated with age-related hearing loss.[29]

### Implications on Aging

Growing evidence demonstrates age-related hearing loss may have important consequences on the aging process. Age-related hearing loss is independently associated with accelerated cognitive decline and incident dementia, in which the degree of risk increases with the severity of hearing loss.[33–44] Given its prevalence and the

**Table 3**
Common causes and recommendations for chronic hearing loss

| Causes of Chronic Hearing Loss | Key History Findings | Key Physical Examination Findings | Treatment |
|---|---|---|---|
| Chronic otitis media +/– cholesteatoma | Chronic purulent otorrhea History of ear infections | Tympanic membrane retraction Keratin debris | Audiogram Consider computed tomography temporal bone without contrast *When to refer:* Nonurgent immediate referral |
| Autoimmune ear disease | History of systemic autoimmune disease Symptom severity mirrors state of systemic disease | Normal otoscopic examination | Systemic treatment of underlying systemic disease Immunosuppressive therapy *When to refer:* If suspected, refer for evaluation, audiogram, treatment planning |
| Vestibular schwannoma | Typically unilateral Progressive or sudden hearing loss +/– Dizziness, vertigo +/– Facial weakness | Normal otoscopic examination +/– Facial paresis/paralysis | MRI brain with gadolinium *When to refer:* Immediate referral |
| Noise-induced hearing loss | Progressive but can be acute +/– Tinnitus History of noise exposure | Normal otoscopic examination | Counsel on hearing protection *When to refer:* Nonurgent immediate referral |
| Age-Related Hearing Loss | Progressive, bilateral hearing loss +/– Tinnitus | Normal otoscopic examination | Communication strategies Amplification: Hearing aid, over-the-counter amplifier, or cochlear implant *When to refer:* Nonurgent immediate referral |

degree of risk, age-related hearing loss is the largest potentially modifiable risk factor for dementia.[33] Age-related hearing loss has also been independently associated with depressive symptoms, anxiety, and loneliness, as well as functional limitations and falls.[45-55]

## Treatment

### Barriers to care and disparities
Multiple barriers to hearing health care exist, including system-level and individual-level factors. The clinic-based hearing health care system in the United States traditionally requires multiples visits to multiple providers and fee-for-service visits not covered by Medicare.[56,57] Only 15% to 20% of older adults with hearing loss use hearing aids, and disparities in care exist based on race/ethnicity and socioeconomic position.[58-61]

### Recent advances in hearing health care
National efforts by leading organizations have translated to major developments in increasing the affordability and accessibility of hearing care, which have been led by the White House President's Council of Advisors on Science and Technology and the National Academies of Sciences, Engineering and Medicine.[57,62,63] As a result of these efforts, in August 2017, a bipartisan bill was signed into law that mandated the Food and Drug Administration (FDA) to create a new regulatory classification for over-the-counter hearing aids within 3 years.[64,65]

## Hearing Aids

### Key components of technology
Hearing aids represent the current gold standard in hearing care. At the most basic level, the hearing aid has 3 components:

1. A microphone to capture sound in the environment
2. An amplifier to process and manipulate sound
3. A receiver to deliver sound to the wearer's ear[66]

### Hearing assistive technologies
Hearing assistive technologies further maximize the capabilities of hearing aids in specific situations.[67] Streaming devices worn as a necklace or clipped on a wearer's lapel can use Bluetooth to send a direct signal from cellular phones to the hearing aids. Remote microphones can be placed by a signal of interest (ie, a fellow diner in a restaurant or at a podium during a speech) and relay a direct signal to a patient's hearing aids.[68] In the home, streaming devices can link signals from televisions and radios directly to the wearer's hearing aids. Remote controls are available to manipulate hearing aid volume and programs as a more practical option for older adults who cannot use the small buttons on the hearing aids themselves.

### Fitting and aural rehabilitation
Hearing aids are adjusted to prescriptive amplification targets and programs are custom designed based on the patient's hearing loss and lifestyle. Equally important as the hearing aid is the counseling and communication strategies that accompany hearing aid fitting (**Table 4**). Often collectively referred to as aural rehabilitation, patients are provided counseling on the use of their device, such as changing batteries, and given strategies to improve communication, such as minimizing background noise (see **Table 4**).[69]

| Table 4 Basic communication strategies for patients with hearing loss | | |
|---|---|---|
| 1 | Rephrase rather than repeat | Rephrasing uses different words that may be easier for the listener to hear depending on their hearing loss and gives new contextual cues for the listener. Repetition can lead to a frustrating loop of miscommunication. |
| 2 | Reduce background noise | Distracting sounds can mask the information that is important for the listener. Understanding speech in the presence of background noise declines as people age, regardless of hearing status. |
| 3 | Visualize the speaker | Good lighting and ensuring face-to-face communication can reduce miscommunication. |
| 4 | Avoid covering your mouth | Whether consciously or not, many people read lips to improve speech understanding. |
| 5 | Give context to the conversation | When the listener knows the topic of conversation, it is easier to use contextual cues to fill in gaps when a word is not heard. |
| 6 | Speak slow, not loud | Hearing loss is often a clarity issue and slowing down can help the listener, whereas shouting can distort language and make it more difficult to understand. |
| 7 | Ensure attention before engaging | The conversation should not start until you are sure everyone is listening, as this can create gaps in context. |

### Over-the-counter options

Personal sound amplification products (PSAPs) represent a potentially affordable and accessible solution for some adults (**Table 5**). PSAPs are unregulated by the FDA and thus not marketed for hearing loss, but recent research suggests some perform technologically similar to hearing aids and improve speech understanding.[70,71] Both ear-level and handheld devices exist. Handheld devices may better serve patients with manual dexterity limitations and/or cognitive impairment.[72] Given the high variability in the PSAP market, see **Table 5** for considerations when buying a PSAP.[70] This market will be further regulated by recent legislation, discussed previously, that requires the FDA to regulate an over-the-counter class of hearing aids for mild to moderate hearing loss by 2020.[64]

### Cochlear Implants

Age-related hearing loss is progressive and, for older adults who have severe to profound hearing loss and no longer benefit from hearing aids, cochlear implantation can be an option.[73,74] Cochlear implantation can benefit adults and older adults and is an outpatient procedure, routinely performed on adults, including octogenarians and nonagenarians.[75] Unlike hearing aids, cochlear implantation is covered by Medicare and most private health insurance. All patients with bilateral severe to profound hearing loss, including older adults, should be referred to an otolaryngologist who performs cochlear implants for evaluation.

**Table 5**
**Checklist of considerations for over-the-counter hearing technology**

| Item | Key Points |
|---|---|
| 1. Battery or rechargeable | Batteries can be costly and difficult to insert when dexterity is an issue; whereas rechargeable devices are easier to manipulate, the user must remember to place the device in the charger regularly |
| 2. Directionality | Devices with directionality can focus on what is in front of the wearer while attempting to ignore distracting sound behind the wearer. This is helpful in noisy environments like a restaurant. |
| 3. Programmable | Programs allow for preset or customized set-ups for various listening environments like a noisy restaurant; this is a helpful feature for an active lifestyle |
| 4. T-coil | T-coils allow users to access a direct signal to the device in "looped" areas with landline telephone usage. However, buildings with looped set-ups are rare, especially in rural areas. |
| 5. Remote microphone | A remote microphone allows a direct signal from a specific sound source to the user. It can be clipped on another person's lapel or set up on a podium. This is especially helpful in presentations or for conversation in a noisy area. |
| 6. Smartphone operated | Smartphone applications may allow for greater control and customization but can be difficult to operate for some older adults |
| 7. User manual | User manuals are often difficult to read and written at high health literacy levels. Devices with picture-based user manuals or available online/video support can be helpful. |
| 8. Specifications | Devices should report their specifications and include frequency range (minimum 250–6000 Hz), internal noise (<24–28 dB), and maximum output (<120 dB sound pressure level). |

## SUMMARY

Numerous conditions can lead to hearing loss, both acutely and over time, and require initial evaluation and otologic examination. Although most causes of hearing loss can be managed initially in a primary care setting, there are a few conditions, such as sudden hearing loss that require urgent treatment and referral. However, the most common cause of hearing loss is age-related hearing loss. With recent advances in technology and legislative changes, affordable and accessible options are increasing and can be offered in an outpatient and direct-to-consumer setting with the appropriate education and counseling.

## REFERENCES

1. Blackwell DL, Lucas JW, Clarke TC. Summary health statistics for U.S. adults: national health interview survey, 2012. Vital Health Stat 10 2014;(260):1–161.
2. Goman AM, Lin FR. Prevalence of hearing loss by severity in the United States. Am J Public Health 2016;106(10):1820–2.
3. Bright T, Pallawela D. Validated smartphone-based apps for ear and hearing assessments: a review. JMIR Rehabil Assist Technol 2016;3(2):e13.

4. Derin S, Cam O, Beydilli H, et al. Initial assessment of hearing loss using a mobile application for audiological evaluation. J Laryngol Otol 2016;130(3):248–51.

5. Thompson GP, Sladen DP, Borst BJH, et al. Accuracy of a tablet audiometer for measuring behavioral hearing thresholds in a clinical population. Otolaryngol Head Neck Surg 2015;153(5):838–42.

6. van Tonder J, Swanepoel DW, Mahomed-Asmail F, et al. Automated smartphone threshold audiometry: validity and time efficiency. J Am Acad Audiol 2017;28(3): 200–8.

7. Burton M, Doree C. Ear drops for the removal of ear wax. Cochrane Database Syst Rev 2003;(3):CD004400.

8. Alberti P. Epithelial migration on the tympanic membrane. J Laryngol Otol 1964; 78(9):808–30.

9. Roland PS, Smith TL, Schwartz SR, et al. Clinical practice guideline: cerumen impaction. Otolaryngol Head Neck Surg 2008;139(3_suppl_1):S1–21.

10. Linstrom CJ, Lucente FE. Diseases of the external ear. In: Johnson JT, Rosen CA, editors. Bailey's head and neck surgery: otolaryngology. 5th edition. Philadelphia: Lippincott Williams & Wilkins; 2014. p. 2333–57.

11. Rosenfeld RM, Schwartz SR, Cannon CR, et al. Clinical practice guideline: acute otitis externa. Otolaryngol Head Neck Surg 2014;150(1_suppl):S1–24.

12. Guss J, Ruckenstein MJ. Infections of the external ear. In: Flint PW, Haughey BH, Lund VJ, et al, editors. Cummings otolaryngology head and neck surgery. 5th edition. Philadelphia: Mosby Elsevier; 2010. p. 1944–9.

13. Davis LE, Johnsson L. Viral infections of the inner ear: clinical, virologic, and pathologic studies in humans and animals. Am J Otolaryngol 1983;4(5):347–62.

14. Vrabec JT, LJ. Acute paralysis of the facial nerve. In: Johnson JT, Rosen CA, editors. Bailey's head and neck surgery: otolaryngology. 5th edition. Philadelphia: Lippincott Williams & Wilkins; 2014. p. 2503–18.

15. Uscategui T, Doree C, Chamberlain IJ, et al. Antiviral therapy for Ramsay Hunt syndrome (herpes zoster oticus with facial palsy) in adults. Cochrane Database Syst Rev 2008;(4):CD006851.

16. Casselbrant ML, Mandel EM. Otitis media in the age of antimicrobial resistance. In: Johnson JT, Rosen CA, editors. Bailey's head and neck surgery: otolaryngology. 5th edition. Philadelphia: Lippincott Williams & Wilkins; 2014. p. 1479–506.

17. Auwaerter PG. Johns Hopkins ABX guide: acute otitis media, adult. 2016. Available at: https://www.hopkinsguides.com/hopkins/view/Johns_Hopkins_ABX_Guide/540408/all/Acute_Otitis_Media_Adult_?q=otitis%20media. Accessed October 4, 2018.

18. Ramakrishnan K, Sparks RA, Berryhill WE. Diagnosis and treatment of otitis media. Am Fam Physician 2007;76(11):1650–8.

19. O'Reilly RC, Sando I. Anatomy and physiology of the eustachian tube. In: Flint PW, Haughey BH, Lund VJ, et al, editors. Cummings otolaryngology head & neck surgery. 5th edition. Philadelphia: Mobsy Elsevier; 2010. p. 1866–75.

20. Syed I, Aldren C. Meniere's disease: an evidence based approach to assessment and management. Int J Clin Pract 2012;66(2):166–70.

21. Sharon JD, Trevino C, Schubert MC, et al. Treatment of Meniere's disease. Curr Treat Options Neurol 2015;17(4):14.

22. Stachler RJ, Chandrasekhar SS, Archer SM, et al. Clinical practice guideline: sudden hearing loss. Otolaryngol Head Neck Surg 2012;146(3_suppl):S1–35.

23. Oliver ER, Hashisaki GT. Sudden sensory hearing loss. In: Johnson JT, Rosen CA, editors. Bailey's head and neck surgery: otolaryngology, vol. 2, 5th edition. Philadelphia: Lippincott Williams & Wilkins; 2014. p. 2589–95.

24. Meyer TA, Strunk CL, Lambert PR. Cholesteatoma. In: Johnson JT, Rosen CA, editors. Bailey's head and neck surgery: otolaryngology, vol. 2, 5th edition. Philadelphia: Lippincott Williams & Wilkins; 2014. p. 2433–46.

25. Chang CYJ. Cholesteatoma. In: Lalwani AK, editor. Current diagnosis and treatment in otolaryngology - head and neck surgery. 3rd edition. New York: McGraw-Hill; 2012. p. 682–8.

26. Roland JT. Autoimmune inner ear disease. Curr Rheumatol Rep 2000;2(2):171–4.

27. Genther DJ, Lin FR. Managing hearing impairment in older adults. In: Williams BA, Chang A, Ahalt C, et al, editors. Current diagnosis & treatment: geriatrics. 2nd edition. New York: McGraw-Hill; 2014. p. 460–7.

28. Lin FR, Niparko JK, Ferrucci L. Hearing loss prevalence in the United States. Arch Intern Med 2011;171(20):1851–3.

29. Lin FR, Thorpe R, Gordon-Salant S, et al. Hearing loss prevalence and risk factors among older adults in the United States. J Gerontol A Biol Sci Med Sci 2011; 66(5):582–90.

30. Helzner EP, Cauley JA, Pratt SR, et al. Race and sex differences in age-related hearing loss: the health, aging and body composition study. J Am Geriatr Soc 2005;53(12):2119–27.

31. Moscicki EK, Elkins EF, Baum HM, et al. Hearing loss in the elderly: an epidemiologic study of the Framingham heart study cohort. Ear Hear 1985;6(4):184–90.

32. Lin FR, Maas P, Chine W, et al. Association of skin color, race/ethnicity, and hearing loss among adults in the USA. J Assoc Res Otolaryngol 2012;13(1):109–17.

33. Livingston G, Sommerlad A, Orgeta V, et al. Dementia prevention, intervention, and care. Lancet 2017;390(10113):2673–734.

34. Lin FR, Metter EJ, O'Brien RJ, et al. Hearing loss and incident dementia. Arch Neurol 2011;68(2):214–20.

35. Gallacher J, Ilubaera V, Ben-Shlomo Y, et al. Auditory threshold, phonologic demand, and incident dementia. Neurology 2012;79(15):1583–90.

36. Lin FR. Hearing loss and cognition among older adults in the United States. J Gerontol A Biol Sci Med Sci 2011;66(10):1131–6.

37. Lin FR, Ferrucci L, Metter EJ, et al. Hearing loss and cognition in the Baltimore longitudinal study of aging. Neuropsychology 2011;25(6):763–70.

38. Deal JA, Sharrett AR, Albert MS, et al. Hearing impairment and cognitive decline: a pilot study conducted within the Atherosclerosis Risk in Communities neurocognitive study. Am J Epidemiol 2015;181(9):680–90.

39. Deal JA, Betz J, Yaffe K, et al. Hearing impairment and incident dementia and cognitive decline in older adults: the health ABC study. Journals Gerontol 2017; 72(5):703–9.

40. Kiely KM, Gopinath B, Mitchell P, et al. Cognitive, health, and sociodemographic predictors of longitudinal decline in hearing acuity among older adults. J Gerontol A Biol Sci Med Sci 2012;67(9):997–1003.

41. Fritze T, Teipel S, Óvári A, et al. Hearing impairment affects dementia incidence. An analysis based on longitudinal health claims data in Germany. PLoS One 2016;11(7):e0156876.

42. Gurgel RK, Ward PD, Schwartz S, et al. Relationship of hearing loss and dementia: a prospective, population-based study. Otol Neurotol 2014;35(5):775–81.

43. Amieva H, Ouvrard C, Giulioli C, et al. Self-reported hearing loss, hearing aids, and cognitive decline in elderly adults: a 25-year study. J Am Geriatr Soc 2015;63(10):2099–104.
44. Valentijn SA, Van Boxtel MP, Van Hooren SA, et al. Change in sensory functioning predicts change in cognitive functioning: results from a 6-year follow-up in the Maastricht aging study. J Am Geriatr Soc 2005;53(3):374–80.
45. Abrams TE, Barnett MJ, Hoth A, et al. The relationship between hearing impairment and depression in older veterans. J Am Geriatr Soc 2006;54(9):1475–7.
46. Monzani D, Galeazzi GM, Genovese E, et al. Psychological profile and social behaviour of working adults with mild or moderate hearing loss. Acta Otorhinolaryngol Ital 2008;28(2):61–6.
47. Gopinath B, Wang JJ, Schneider J, et al. Depressive symptoms in older adults with hearing impairments: the Blue Mountains Study. J Am Geriatr Soc 2009; 57(7):1306–8.
48. Mener DJ, Betz J, Genther DJ, et al. Hearing loss and depression in older adults. J Am Geriatr Soc 2013;61(9):1627–9.
49. Huang C, Dong B, Lu Z, et al. Chronic diseases and risk for depression in old age: a meta-analysis of published literature. Ageing Res Rev 2010;9(2):131–41.
50. Contrera KJ, Betz J, Deal J, et al. Association of hearing impairment and anxiety in older adults. J Aging Health 2017;29(1):172–84.
51. Sung Y, Li L, Blake C, et al. Association of hearing loss and loneliness in older adults. J Aging Health 2016;28(6):979–94.
52. Pronk M, Deeg DJ, Smits C, et al. Prospective effects of hearing status on loneliness and depression in older persons: identification of subgroups. Int J Audiol 2011;50(12):887–96.
53. Lin FR, Ferrucci L. Hearing loss and falls among older adults in the United States. Arch Intern Med 2012;172(4):369–71.
54. Viljanen A, Kaprio J, Pyykkö I, et al. Hearing as a predictor of falls and postural balance in older female twins. J Gerontol A Biol Sci Med Sci 2009;64(2):312–7.
55. Dalton DS, Cruickshanks KJ, Klein BE, et al. The impact of hearing loss on quality of life in older adults. Gerontologist 2003;43(5):661–8.
56. Valente M, Abrams H, Benson D, et al. Guidelines for the audiologic management of adult hearing impairment. Audiol Today 2006;18(5):32–7.
57. National Academies of Sciences, Engineering, and Medicine. Hearing health care for adults: Priorities for improving access and affordability. Washington, DC: The National Academies Press; 2016.
58. Nieman CL, Marrone N, Szanton SL, et al. Racial/ethnic and socioeconomic disparities in hearing health care among older Americans. J Aging Health 2016; 28(1):68–94.
59. Mamo SK, Nieman CL, Lin FR. Prevalence of untreated hearing loss by income among older adults in the United States. J Health Care Poor Underserved 2016;27(4):1812–8.
60. Bainbridge KE, Ramachandran V. Hearing aid use among older U.S. adults; the National Health and Nutrition Examination Survey, 2005-2006 and 2009-2010. Ear Hear 2014;35(3):289–94.
61. Chien W, Lin FR. Prevalence of hearing aid use among older adults in the United States. Arch Intern Med 2012;172(3):292–3.
62. Nieman CL, Lin FR. Increasing access to hearing rehabilitation for older adults. Curr Opin Otolaryngol Head Neck Surg 2017;25(5):342–6.
63. President's Council of Advisors on Science and Technology (PCAST). Aging America & hearing loss: Imperative of improved hearing technologies. 2015.

Available at: https://www.whitehouse.gov/sites/default/files/microsites/ostp/PCAST/pcast_hearing_tech_letterreport_final.pdf. Accessed March 11, 2016.

64. Warren E, Grassley C. Over-the-counter hearing aids: the path forward. JAMA Intern Med 2017;177(5):609–10.

65. Rep. Greg Walden. Congress US. HR 2430: FDA Reauthorization Act of 2017. August 29, 2017.

66. Dillon H. Hearing aids. New York: Hodder Arnold; 2008.

67. Chisolm TH, Noe CM, McArdle R, et al. Evidence for the use of hearing assistive technology by adults: the role of the FM system. Trends Amplif 2007;11(2):73–89.

68. Hartley D, Rochtchina E, Newall P, et al. Use of hearing aids and assistive listening devices in an older Australian population. J Am Acad Audiol 2010; 21(10):642–53.

69. Boothroyd A. Adult aural rehabilitation: what is it and does it work? Trends Amplif 2007;11(2):63–71.

70. Reed NS, Betz J, Lin FR, et al. Pilot electroacoustic analyses of a sample of direct-to-consumer amplification products. Otol Neurotol 2017;38(6):804–8.

71. Reed NS, Betz J, Kendig N, et al. Personal sound amplification products vs a conventional hearing aid for speech understanding in noise. JAMA 2017; 318(1):89–90.

72. Mamo SK, Reed NS, Nieman CL, et al. Personal sound amplifiers for adults with hearing loss. Am J Med 2016;129(3):245.

73. Sprinzl GM, Riechelmann H. Current trends in treating hearing loss in elderly people: a review of the technology and treatment options - a mini-review. Gerontology 2010;56(3):351–8.

74. Chen DS, Clarrett DM, Li L, et al. Cochlear implantation in older adults: long-term analysis of complications and device survival in a consecutive series. Otol Neurotol 2013;34(7):1272–7.

75. Carlson ML, Breen JT, Gifford RH, et al. Cochlear implantation in the octogenarian and nonagenarian. Otol Neurotol 2010;31(8):1343–9.

# Sinuses and Common Rhinologic Conditions

Nyall R. London Jr, MD, PhD, Murugappan Ramanathan Jr, MD*

## KEYWORDS

• Allergic rhinitis • Acute rhinosinusitis • Chronic rhinosinusitis • Epistaxis

## KEY POINTS

- Epistaxis predominantly arises from an anterior nasal source and is often controlled with gentle finger pressure and oxymetazoline. Preventive measures may be used to limit recurrent epistaxis episodes.
- Allergic rhinitis is an immunoglobulin E–mediated disease of the nasal cavity resulting from exposure of the sinonasal cavity to inhaled allergens. Symptoms include rhinorrhea, congestion, sneezing, and nasal itching, and empiric first-line therapy includes intranasal steroid sprays.
- Acute rhinosinusitis is defined as nasal congestion, purulent rhinorrhea, facial pain/pressure, and change in sense of smell of less than a 4-week duration and often arises from an acute viral or bacterial cause.
- Chronic rhinosinusitis presents with similar symptoms but of greater than 12-week duration. Underlying dysregulated inflammatory pathways are at the center of chronic rhinosinusitis, and treatment focuses on means of reducing sinonasal inflammation, including nasal saline irrigations, corticosteroids, and prolonged antibiotics.

## INTRODUCTION

Some of the most common rhinologic disorders that may present to the primary care provider include disorders of hemostasis, such as epistaxis, or sinonasal inflammatory disorders, such as allergic rhinitis and acute (ARS) or chronic rhinosinusitis (CRS). Management of these conditions varies greatly. The goal for epistaxis is to control active bleeding, elicit the underlying cause, and offer preventive strategies to prevent future episodes, often targeting reducing nasal dryness. Allergic rhinitis is an immunoglobulin G (IgE) -mediated disease characterized by rhinorrhea, congestion, sneezing, and nasal itching from allergen exposure. First-line treatment includes avoiding known allergic triggers and intranasal steroid sprays. ARS and CRS are characterized by

Disclosures: The authors declare no relevant conflicts of interest.
Department of Otolaryngology–Head and Neck Surgery, Johns Hopkins University School of Medicine, 601 North Caroline Street, 6th Floor, Baltimore, MD 21287, USA
* Corresponding author. Department of Otolaryngology–Head and Neck Surgery, Johns Hopkins Outpatient Center, 601 North Caroline Street, 6th Floor, 6263, Baltimore, MD 21287.
E-mail address: mramana3@jhmi.edu

similar symptoms, including nasal congestion, purulent rhinorrhea, facial pain/pressure, and change in sense of smell, but differ in duration of less than 4 weeks or greater than 12 weeks, respectively. Management for ARS from viral cause centers on symptom management, whereas uncomplicated bacterial sinusitis may include observation versus treatment with antibiotics. CRS in contrast is characterized by dysregulation of underlying inflammatory pathways, and management centers on control of sinonasal inflammation. This article is written with the intent to review and summarize these common rhinologic conditions for primary care providers.

## EPISTAXIS
### Symptoms

Epistaxis is often a self-limiting event that 60% of individuals experience at some point during their life.[1] The degree of epistaxis one may experience however ranges from minor bleeding requiring little intervention to life-threatening hemorrhage. The variance in hemorrhage may depend on multiple factors, including the origin of bleeding, as well as multiple patient comorbidities, such as hypertension, thrombocytopenia, anticoagulation, underlying vascular malformations/tumors, and concurrent medication use, such as steroid nasal sprays.[2,3] Greater than 90% of nosebleeds originate in the anterior nasal cavity.[4] On the nasal septum, there is a convergence of multiple arterial supplies known as Kisselbach plexus. Epistaxis arising from an anterior source may be much more straightforward to control than a posterior nosebleed arising from the sphenopalatine artery posterior blood supply.[2,5] When evaluating a patient for epistaxis, it is important to take a thorough history and characterize the episode or episodes of epistaxis with details, such as degree of bleeding, frequency, laterality, and any resultant symptoms, such as lightheadedness or syncope.

### Diagnostic Testing

The decision to perform diagnostic testing, if any, is predicated upon the story, physical examination findings, and contributory medical history. On presentation to the primary care provider, diagnostic analysis should include obtaining vital signs whereby tachycardia or hypotension may demonstrate disease severity or urgency for intervention. Hypertension, however, has been associated with epistaxis on meta-analysis, and adequate control of hypertension may help to reduce active epistaxis in some patients as well as prevent future episodes.[6] Next, one should consider anterior rhinoscopy to examine the nasal cavities and distinguish the origin of the epistaxis. Furthermore, the primary care provider may consider obtaining a hemoglobin/hematocrit level, especially if the bleeding was severe or the patient had been symptomatic. Additional diagnostic testing may include coagulation studies for patients on anticoagulants or for concern for a bleeding disorder.[3] Radiographic studies generally are not indicated as routine diagnostic work-up for epistaxis.

### Differential Diagnosis

The differential diagnosis of causes of epistaxis is vast. The most common cause of epistaxis is trauma from digital manipulation.[5] Additional sources of trauma include fractures or drying of nasal mucosa from air delivered via nasal cannula or exposure to nonhumidified environments. Use of intranasal steroid sprays is also well known to contribute to epistaxis.[7,8] Furthermore, the technique whereby patients apply nasal spray may also contribute to increased episodes of epistaxis. Additional causes of epistaxis include nasal masses or malignancies, anticoagulative medication or inherited coagulopathies, and platelet abnormalities.[2] Keeping a broad differential diagnosis in regards to the cause of epistaxis may aid in reversal of active bleeding as well as enacting means to prevent future episodes.

### Management/Treatment

Initial management and treatment of epistaxis are predicated on first stopping active bleeding. As previously mentioned, greater than 90% of episodes originate anteriorly. Therefore, gentle finger pressure should be applied to pinch the cartilaginous nasal tip so as to apply pressure to the anterior nasal septum. Finger pressure should be performed for an adequate duration to achieve hemostasis and may take 15 to 20 minutes. One may also consider an icepack for initial first aid management, although there is not strong evidence of efficacy.[3] If oxymetazoline is available and there are no contraindications, this may be sprayed into the nasal cavity to aid in vasoconstriction and achieving hemostasis. Oxymetazoline also acts as a decongestant and should not be used for more than 72 hours to prevent rebound congestion. The use of gentle finger pressure and oxymetazoline is adequate to stop most epistaxis.

For epistaxis refractory to these initial management strategies, one may consider anterior nasal packing. Anterior nasal packing is often left in place for 2 to 3 days before removal along with antibiotic administration for Staphylococcus coverage while the packing is in place. Depending on the cause of epistaxis, control of hypertension or reversal of anticoagulation or correction of platelet abnormalities if applicable may also aid in achieving hemostasis. More aggressive interventions for control of epistaxis are outside the scope of this article. After achieving hemostasis, it is important to consider the cause of the epistaxis so that preventive measures may be considered, including nasal saline sprays, humidification, and nighttime nasal moisturizers such as Ayr gel. The authors typically avoid intranasal application of petrolatum ointment as a nasal moisturizer because of reports of the development of exogenous lipoid pneumonia.[9] During the management and treatment process, one should also consider the applicability of Otolaryngology consultation or referral.[10] Referral to an Otolaryngologist is particularly important in the setting of recurrent epistaxis so that nasal endoscopy may be performed to rule out more sinister causes of epistaxis. There have yet to be national guidelines developed for epistaxis, although the American Academy of Otolaryngology Head and Neck Surgery (AAO-HNS) has announced guidelines to come in June 2019.[3,11]

## ALLERGIC RHINITIS
### Symptoms

Allergic rhinitis is an IgE-mediated disease of the nasal cavity resulting from exposure of the sinonasal cavity to allergens.[12] Symptoms resulting from these exposures include rhinorrhea, congestion, sneezing, and nasal itching.[13–15] Allergic rhinitis is very common and estimated to affect 1 in 6 Americans.[14] Some of the most common allergens include house dust mite antigen, pollen, environmental exposures, and animal dander.[15] Allergic rhinitis can be divided based on the duration and degree of symptoms. Patients may suffer from symptoms year round (perennial), seasonally, and episodically. Symptoms can be further classified as intermittent (less than 4 days a week or 4 weeks per year) or persistent (more than 4 days a week or 4 weeks per year).[13,14] Severity may be further distinguished as mild if there is no impingement on quality of life or severe if impairment in quality of life is apparent.[14]

### Diagnostic Testing

Before initiating any diagnostic testing, a primary care provider should first take a complete history and perform a physical examination. The history should include characterizing the symptoms, duration, and impact on quality of life as well as discussion of any known triggers. Symptoms that may suggest an alternative diagnosis than allergic rhinitis should also be elicited during the patient encounter. These findings may include epistaxis, anosmia, cranial nerve deficits, and unilateral nature of rhinorrhea.[14] Anterior rhinoscopy should also be performed during the physical examination. Although referral to an allergist for allergy testing may be beneficial, this is typically reserved for patients with an uncertain diagnosis or those who do not respond to empiric therapy.[14] Skin prick testing may be performed by an allergist to ascertain specific allergic response to a battery of common perennial, seasonal, and episodic exposures. Imaging is also typically not recommended for a diagnosis of allergic rhinitis but may be considered if alternative diagnoses are considered. Referral to an Otolaryngologist may also be considered for nasal endoscopy and direct visualization of the nasal mucosa or if an alternative diagnosis is suspected.

### Differential Diagnosis

There are many conditions that mimic symptoms found in allergic rhinitis. As previously mentioned, these alternative diagnoses should be considered if atypical symptoms are present. A cerebrospinal fluid leak should be considered if rhinorrhea is present unilaterally, especially with a history of previous sinus surgery or recent trauma. There is overlap and concurrent nature between patients with allergic rhinitis as well as other chronic sinonasal inflammatory conditions, such as CRS. If the patient endorses symptoms including facial pain/pressure or loss of sense of smell, one should also consider a diagnosis of CRS. In addition to allergic IgE-mediated sinonasal inflammation, there are a multitude of additional possible causes of rhinorrhea, nasal congestion, and nasal itching termed nonallergic rhinitis. Some of these include drug-induced, rhinitis medicamentosa, occupational, infectious, pregnancy/hormone-related, gustatory, nonallergic rhinitis with eosinophilia syndrome, vasomotor rhinitis, or autoimmune related.[13,16,17] Thus, when taking a patient history, it is also important to consider nonallergic causes of rhinitis.

### Management/Treatment

When a diagnosis of allergic rhinitis is made and the allergen is known, the first step in management may be avoidance of allergen exposure. In many cases, however, this is challenging for patients to adhere to. For example, although removal of pets from the household may be beneficial for patients with an allergy to animal dander, many patients are reluctant to do so.[14] Additional approaches that may reduce allergen exposures include air filtration systems or allergen impermeable bed covers[14]; however, these measures may or may not be efficacious in symptom management. Empiric medical therapy is indicated for patients with symptoms that affect quality of life. According to AAO-HNS guidelines, the first-line treatment is intranasal steroids. It is important to inform patients initiating intranasal steroid use that it may take weeks to demonstrate efficacy and that these sprays should be used on a daily rather than intermittent basis to achieve maximum benefit.[14] The most common side effects from intranasal steroid use are epistaxis and nasal dryness. Oral second-generation or intranasal antihistamines are generally reserved for patients with nasal itching and sneezing. Patients who do not respond to empiric therapy should be referred to an allergist for allergen testing. Additional treatment approaches, including subcutaneous or sublingual immunotherapy, may be considered by an allergist for long-term symptom control.[13,18]

## ACUTE AND CHRONIC RHINOSINUSITIS
### Symptoms

Rhinosinusitis is common and can affect up to 1 in 8 adults.[19] ARS is defined as nasal congestion, purulent rhinorrhea, facial pain/pressure, and change in sense of smell of less than a 4-week duration.[19,20] In contrast, CRS symptoms are present for greater than 12 weeks. Despite the similar set of symptoms, the pathophysiology of ARS often arises from infectious cause (viral or bacterial) and may be influenced by predisposing factors, including anatomic allergic and environmental factors, whereas CRS is regarded as dysregulated endogenous Th1- or Th2-mediated inflammatory pathways. CRS has been further subdivided in the past into 2 main groups dependent on the absence of nasal polyps or presence of nasal polyps. Despite this simplification, the pathophysiology is far more complex, and further clusters known as "endotypes" have recently been described.[21] These endotype clusters are based on correlation of inflammatory cytokines, including interleukin-5, and biomarkers, such as IgE, and albumin concentrations with phenotypes including the presence of polyps and asthma. The hypothesis is that subdividing patients into endotypes will help develop and identify targeted therapies for patients suffering across the spectrum of CRS pathophysiology. Another concept in sinonasal inflammatory pathologic condition popularized over the past several decades is the unified airway.[22] Overlap has been noted between upper sinonasal inflammatory disease such as rhinitis and CRS and inflammatory disease of the lower airway (asthma). These diseases often occur concurrently, and exacerbation of upper airway sinonasal disease may negatively impact lower airway inflammatory disease and vice versa.[22–24] Thus, patients who present to the primary care provider with sinonasal inflammatory symptoms may also be suffering from asthma.[25]

### Diagnostic Testing

The diagnosis of ARS is largely clinical and supported by a complete history and physical examination with correlation of sinonasal symptoms.[20] Anterior rhinoscopy to examine the nasal mucosa may also aid in diagnosis. Additional diagnostic testing is often not necessary in uncomplicated cases.[20] However, imaging techniques should be considered when ocular or intracranial complications of ARS are suspected.[20,26,27] One challenge with ARS for the primary care provider whereby nasal endoscopy is not immediately available is diagnostically distinguishing between ARS arising from a viral or bacterial cause. In this setting, ARS is often assumed to arise from a bacterial cause if symptom duration is greater than 7 to 10 days or if there is a period of improvement followed by worsening of symptoms.[20,28] Unilateral localized pain has also been proposed as a potential signal of bacterial cause, although this is not widely accepted.[20]

Obtaining a diagnosis of CRS is challenging in the absence of nasal endoscopy and computed tomographic (CT) imaging studies. A patient who has not responded to empiric treatment measures by the primary care provider should be referred to an Otolaryngologist so nasal endoscopy can be performed. Although anterior rhinoscopy can reveal mucopurulent drainage or nasal polyposis, nasal endoscopy can allow for improved visualization as well as the ability to obtain site-directed cultures.[20] Typically an Otolaryngologist will obtain a sinus CT scan after trial of maximum medical therapy to ascertain the presence of radiographic mucosal changes resistant to medical therapy.

### Differential Diagnosis

Multiple diseases mimic aspects of rhinosinusitis and should be included on the differential diagnosis for ARS and CRS, including allergic rhinitis, dental disease, facial pain syndromes, and headache.[20] Although allergic rhinitis can also be characterized by nasal congestion and rhinorrhea, often the onset occurs with allergen exposure, and facial pressure/pain is uncommon. Many types of headache are known, including tension, migraine, and cluster headache, and should thus be considered when evaluating a patient for "sinus" headache. Orofacial pain syndromes[20] should also be considered; however, these patients will frequently be lacking of other characteristics of rhinosinusitis. The differential diagnosis when evaluating patients who present with nasal obstruction, facial pain, and a nasal mass is also vast and includes nasal polyps, inverted papilloma, antrochoanal polyp, encephalocele, and multiple tumors, such as esthesioneuroblastoma, lymphoma, and squamous cell carcinoma.[29] A heightened awareness should be maintained when the mass is unilateral or if there are associated cranial neuropathies.

### Management/Treatment

The management of ARS depends on whether the cause is viral or bacterial. Viral rhinosinusitis is very common, generally resolves within 2 weeks, and can be associated with cough, sore throat, rhinorrhea, and nasal congestion.[19] Viral rhinosinusitis is often self-limiting but may progress to secondary bacterial infection in a small number of cases. Initial management of viral rhinosinusitis centers on symptom management, including analgesics, decongestants, nasal saline irrigation, and consideration of intranasal steroids.[19] According to guidelines for uncomplicated acute bacterial rhinosinusitis, a provider should either prescribe antibiotics or offer observation if there is assurance of follow-up whereby antibiotics may be initiated if the condition fails to improve 7 days after diagnosis or if their condition worsens.[19] If antibiotics are initiated, according to guidelines, amoxicillin with or without clavulanate should be used for 5 to 10 days in most adults.[19] Surgery for patients with acute bacterial rhinosinusitis is often reserved for patients with complications from infections or found to have an anatomic abnormality contributing to recurrent episodes.

The management of CRS differs from ARS because of differences in pathophysiology. As CRS is based on underlying dysregulation of inflammatory pathways, treatment is centered on means of controlling sinonasal inflammation.[30] One common treatment of CRS is nasal saline irrigation. Use of nasal saline irrigations, which may be performed several times per day, has been reported to improve quality-of-life scores.[20] The risks and side effects of nasal saline irrigations are minimal; however, the patient must use sterile or distilled saline because cases of primary amebic meningoencephalitis have been reported from the use of contaminated water.[31] Control of sinonasal inflammation can often be achieved with a course of oral corticosteroids. However, multiple side effects, including gastrointestinal complaints, weight gain, and dysregulation of blood sugar levels, among others, limit the duration and frequency of oral corticosteroid use. Maximum medical therapy also includes several weeks of an antibiotic with anti-inflammatory properties. Additional therapeutic options include intranasal administration of steroids via either nasal steroid sprays or Budesonide rinses. Surgery is generally reserved for patients resistant to maximum medical therapy. Endoscopic sinus surgery allows for opening of sinonasal passages to improve intranasal administration of steroid rinses.

### REFERENCES

1. Murray S, Mendez A, Hopkins A, et al. Management of persistent epistaxis using floseal hemostatic matrix vs. traditional nasal packing: a prospective randomized control trial. J Otolaryngol Head Neck Surg 2018;47(1). https://doi.org/10.1186/s40463-017-0248-5.

2. Sacks R, Sacks PL, Chandra R. Chapter 3: epistaxis. Am J Rhinol Allergy 2013; 27(3):9–10.

3. Khan M, Conroy K, Ubayasiri K, et al. Initial assessment in the management of adult epistaxis: systematic review. J Laryngol Otol 2017;131(12):1035–55.

4. Douglas R, Wormald PJ. Update on epistaxis. Curr Opin Otolaryngol Head Neck Surg 2007;15(3):180–3.

5. Morgan DJ, Kellerman R. Epistaxis: evaluation and treatment. Prim Care 2014; 41(1):63–73.

6. Min HJ, Kang H, Choi GJ, et al. Association between hypertension and epistaxis: systematic review and meta-analysis. Otolaryngol Head Neck Surg 2017;157(6): 921–7.

7. Benninger MS. Epistaxis and its relationship to handedness with use of intranasal steroid spray. Ear Nose Throat J 2008;87(8):463–5.

8. Ganesh V, Banigo A, McMurran AEL, et al. Does intranasal steroid spray technique affect side effects and compliance? Results of a patient survey. J Laryngol Otol 2017;131(11):991–6.

9. Kilaru H, Prasad S, Radha S, et al. Nasal application of petrolatum ointment - A silent cause of exogenous lipoid pneumonia: successfully treated with prednisolone. Respir Med Case Rep 2017;22:98–100.

10. Shargorodsky J, Bleier BS, Holbrook EH, et al. Outcomes analysis in epistaxis management: development of a therapeutic algorithm. Otolaryngol Head Neck Surg 2013;149(3):390–8.

11. Clinical Practice Guideline: Epistaxis n.d. Available at: http://www.entnet.org/ Clinical%20Practice%20Guideline%3A%20Epistaxis. Accessed April 17, 2018.

12. London NR, Tharakan A, Lane AP, et al. Nuclear erythroid 2-related factor 2 activation inhibits house dust mite-induced sinonasal epithelial cell barrier dysfunction: house dust mite and Nrf2 activation. Int Forum Allergy Rhinol 2017;7(5): 536–41.

13. Wise SK, Lin SY, Toskala E, et al. International consensus statement on allergy and rhinology: allergic rhinitis: ICAR: allergic rhinitis. Int Forum Allergy Rhinol 2018;8(2):108–352.

14. Seidman MD, Gurgel RK, Lin SY, et al. Clinical practice guideline: allergic rhinitis. Otolaryngol Head Neck Surg 2015;152(1_suppl):S1–43.

15. London NR, Ramanathan M. The role of the sinonasal epithelium in allergic rhinitis. Otolaryngol Clin North Am 2017;50(6):1043–50.

16. Ramanathan M, London NR, Tharakan A, et al. Airborne particulate matter induces nonallergic eosinophilic sinonasal inflammation in mice. Am J Respir Cell Mol Biol 2017;57(1):59–65.

17. Settipane RA, Kaliner MA. Chapter 14: nonallergic rhinitis. Am J Rhinol Allergy 2013;27(3):48–51.

18. Mims JW. Advancements and dilemmas in the management of allergy. Otolaryngol Clin North Am 2017;50(6):1037–42.

19. Rosenfeld RM, Piccirillo JF, Chandrasekhar SS, et al. Clinical practice guideline (update): adult sinusitis. Otolaryngol Head Neck Surg 2015;152(2_suppl):S1–39.

20. Orlandi RR, Kingdom TT, Hwang PH, et al. International consensus statement on allergy and rhinology: rhinosinusitis: international consensus on rhinosinusitis. Int Forum Allergy Rhinol 2016;6(S1):S22–209.

21. Tomassen P, Vandeplas G, Van Zele T, et al. Inflammatory endotypes of chronic rhinosinusitis based on cluster analysis of biomarkers. J Allergy Clin Immunol 2016;137(5):1449–56.e4.

22. Stachler RJ. Comorbidities of asthma and the unified airway: comorbidities of asthma and the unified airway. Int Forum Allergy Rhinol 2015;5(S1):S17–22.

23. John Staniorski C, Price CPE, Weibman AR, et al. Asthma onset pattern and patient outcomes in a chronic rhinosinusitis population: asthma onset and patient characteristics in CRS. Int Forum Allergy Rhinol 2018;8(4):495–503.

24. Bachert C, Claeys SEM, Tomassen P, et al. Rhinosinusitis and asthma: a link for asthma severity. Curr Allergy Asthma Rep 2010;10(3):194–201.

25. Frendø M, Håkansson K, Schwer S, et al. Asthma in ear, nose, and throat primary care patients with chronic rhinosinusitis with nasal polyps. Am J Rhinol Allergy 2016;30(3):67–71.

26. Jabarin B, Eviatar E, Israel O, et al. Indicators for imaging in periorbital cellulitis secondary to rhinosinusitis. Eur Arch Otorhinolaryngol 2018;275(4):943–8.

27. Kirsch CFE, Bykowski J, Aulino JM, et al. ACR appropriateness criteria ® sinonasal disease. J Am Coll Radiol 2017;14(11):S550–9.

28. van den Broek MFM, Gudden C, Kluijfhout WP, et al. No evidence for distinguishing bacterial from viral acute rhinosinusitis using symptom duration and purulent rhinorrhea: a systematic review of the evidence base. Otolaryngol Head Neck Surg 2014;150(4):533–7.

29. London NR Jr, Reh DD. Differential diagnosis of chronic rhinosinusitis with nasal polyps. In: Woodworth BA, Poetker DM, Reh DD, editors. Advances in oto-rhino-laryngology, vol. 79. Basel (Switzerland): S. Karger AG; 2016. p. 1–12.

30. London NR, Lane AP. Innate immunity and chronic rhinosinusitis: what we have learned from animal models: innate immunity and CRS. Laryngoscope Investig Otolaryngol 2016;1(3):49–56.

31. Yoder JS, Straif-Bourgeois S, Roy SL, et al. Primary amebic Meningoencephalitis deaths associated with sinus irrigation using contaminated tap water. Clin Infect Dis 2012;55(9):e79–85.

# Dizziness and the Otolaryngology Point of View

Sharmeen Sorathia[a,b], Yuri Agrawal, MD, MPH[c],
Michael C. Schubert, PT PhD[c,d],*

## KEYWORDS

- Dizziness • Vertigo • Evaluation • Physical therapy • History • Examination
- Vestibular tests

## KEY POINTS

- Dizziness can be classified as vertigo, lightheadedness, oscillopsia, or disequilibrium. It is most commonly caused by peripheral vestibular disorders.
- Vertigo is an illusion of motion often caused by asymmetric stimulation of the vestibular pathway. It is most common in benign paroxysmal positional vertigo (BPPV), Meniere disease, and vestibular neuritis.
- Evaluation of dizziness from the otolaryngology point of view includes essential components in the history, examination, and vestibular function tests.
- Vestibular rehabilitation plays an integral role in the management of vertigo. For BPPV, the classic treatment is canalith repositioning maneuvers.

## INTRODUCTION
### Dizziness and Its Types

Dizziness is a broad term used to describe several sensations that are typically categorized as vertigo, disequilibrium, lightheadedness, or oscillopsia.

It is a commonly reported symptom presenting to specialists and emergency departments affecting 15% to 20% of the general adult population.[1,2] It is reported to be more prevalent in women and the elderly.[1]

Disclosure Statement: None of the authors have any disclosure.
[a] Ziauddin University College of Medicine, 4/B, Shahrah-e-Ghalib, Block 6, Clifton, Karachi 75600, Pakistan; [b] Johns Hopkins University School of Medicine, 601 North Caroline Street, Baltimore, MD 21287, USA; [c] Department of Otolaryngology–Head and Neck Surgery, Johns Hopkins University School of Medicine, 601 North Caroline Street, Baltimore, MD 21287, USA; [d] Department of Physical Medicine and Rehabilitation, Johns Hopkins University School of Medicine, 601 North Caroline Street, Baltimore, MD 21287, USA
* Corresponding author. Johns Hopkins University School of Medicine, 601 North Caroline Street, Baltimore, MD 21287.
E-mail address: mschube1@jhmi.edu

Med Clin N Am 102 (2018) 1001–1012
https://doi.org/10.1016/j.mcna.2018.06.004
0025-7125/18/© 2018 Elsevier Inc. All rights reserved.

It can be caused by a disturbance in multiple systems or pathways, including the central nervous system (CNS) and the vestibular end organ, but also the visual pathways, the cardiovascular system, and others. It can also have an association with anxiety and panic disorder. Because of the symptoms being vague and the large number of causes for dizziness, the clinical diagnosis and management can be challenging.

### Common Causes

The nonspecific symptom of dizziness can have numerous causes ranging from life-threatening to benign conditions. A critical review from 12 studies conducted on the cause of dizziness classifies and reports the quality-adjusted[a] mean frequencies of various causes, summarized in **Table 1**.[3] The most common classifications are peripheral vestibular conditions followed by nonvestibular and nonpsychotic, psychiatric, unknown, and central vestibular causes.

Vertigo is the sense of spinning or an illusion of a movement that is often described as being objective (ie, the world is moving) or subjective (the person feels as if they are moving). It is caused by an asymmetrical stimulation of the vestibular pathway and thus can be due to intrinsic peripheral or central vestibular diseases or external contributors that affect the pathway (ie, neurologic disease, medication). Common

| Table 1<br>Causes of dizziness | |
| --- | --- |
| **Cause** | **Mean Frequency (%)** |
| Peripheral vestibular | 44 |
|   Benign paroxysmal positional vertigo | 16 |
|   Labyrinthitis | 9 |
|   Meniere disease | 5 |
|   Other (drug-related ototoxicity or nonspecific) | 14 |
| Central vestibular | 11 |
|   Cerebrovascular | 6 |
|   Tumor | <1 |
|   Other (multiple sclerosis, migraine, or other) | 3 |
| Psychiatric | 16 |
|   Psychiatric disorder | 11 |
|   Hyperventilation | 5 |
| Nonvestibular, nonpsychotic | 26 |
|   Presyncope | 6 |
|   Disequilibrium | 5 |
|   Other (anemia, metabolic, drug-related, Parkinson, and other) | 13 |
| Unknown | 13 |

The percentages add up to more than 100% due to dizziness being attributed to more than one cause in some patients.

*Data from* Kroenke K, Hoffman RM, Einstadter D. How common are various causes of dizziness? A Critical Review. South Med J 2000;93(2):162; with permission.

---

[a] Quality adjusted: square root of the study's quality score to enable weighting of the means of each study.

peripheral vestibular diseases include benign paroxysmal positional vertigo (BPPV), Meniere disease, and vestibular neuritis.

Lightheadedness is defined as a sensation of about to faint. Causes of lightheadedness include cardiovascular disease, including cardiac arrhythmias, orthostatic hypotension, hypoglycemia, and anxiety. Orthostatic hypotension is a common cause of lightheadedness.

Disequilibrium is the impairment in balance or coordination such that confident ambulation is disturbed. It can be due to decreased somatosensation or weakness in the lower extremities, but also due to peripheral or central vestibular disorders, multiple sensory deficits, transient ischemic attacks (TIA), or Parkinson disease.

Oscillopsia is defined as the illusion of motion of objects known to be stationary in the visual surround. It is typically caused by loss of vestibular sensation.

## THE CLINICAL EVALUATION OF THE VESTIBULAR SYSTEM
### History

It is essential to take a thorough history of a patient presenting with a complaint of dizziness. A detailed description could reveal the sensation to be of spinning of one's self or surroundings (or both), feeling of about to fall, or becoming out of balance or experiencing motion of stationary objects in the surrounding. The vertigo can be described by the patient as a feeling of rotating, swaying, or falling.[4] Recent studies suggest that the quality of the dizziness symptom may be less informative than the timing, frequency, and triggers of symptoms.[5]

### Episodes and duration
It is critical to inquire about the duration and the temporal characteristic of the vertigo (ie, episodic or constant). Chronic episodic vertigo could indicate BPPV, Meniere disease, or vestibular migraine. BPPV episodes tend to be recurrent and typically occur within 1 minute. In contrast, vestibular migraine and TIA tend to cause single episodes with vertigo durations from minutes to hours. Meniere's disease typically presents with recurrent attacks (2 or more) lasting for 20 minutes to 12 hours. A severe attack of acute spontaneous vertigo for the first time lasting 24 hours or longer is most commonly due to vestibular neuritis. It could also be due to a cerebellar infarct.

### Position
Positional changes are distinctive of BPPV and typically occur upon lying down, rolling over in bed, or bending over/reaching up. These patients tend to not have any vertigo at rest. Occasionally, vestibular migraine could also manifest with positional vertigo, although the duration is commonly longer. Orthostatic hypotension can occur when the patient arises upright from supine or sitting positions, although this does not tend to cause a spinning sensation. Typically, episodes of vertigo due to vestibular migraine, Meniere disease, vestibular neuritis, and TIA occur spontaneously without positional changes.

### Association
Attacks of Meniere are classically associated with hearing loss, aural fullness, and tinnitus, which will be located to one ear. There can also be associated nausea, vomiting, visual disturbance, anxiety, and/or motion sensitivity. Central pathologic conditions are usually associated with severe imbalance, problems with oculomotor control, ataxia, seizures, nausea, and other neurologic symptoms. In particular, hearing impairment is usually caused by Meniere disease or labyrinthitis, whereas vertigo in

BPPV or vestibular neuritis is not associated with hearing loss. Although headaches may or may not be prominent in vestibular migraine, motion sensitivity, photophobia, phonophobia, aura, and nausea are common.

***Others including drugs, social, recent events, impact on daily life***
BPPV mostly frequently occurs in the middle aged and elderly.[2,6,7] Patients should be asked if their symptoms are experienced while driving or riding in vehicles, traveling with public transportation, or during the routine activities of daily life. Depression and anxiety should be addressed because unique surroundings such as supermarkets or crowded spaces can create symptoms of dizziness and imbalance. Recent medical events should be assessed. For example, the onset of an antihypertensive medication might be causing orthostatic hypotension, or a recent head trauma might have preceded BPPV. Alcohol, nicotine, and caffeine can all potentially aggravate vertiginous symptoms.[8,9] Current or previous use of medications should be taken into account. Aminoglycosides, furosemide, ethacrynic acid, acetylsalicylic acid, amiodarone, quinine, and cisplatin can all lead to ototoxicity.[8,10] Sexual history should also be investigated because some sexually transmitted diseases (ie, syphilis) can manifest in vestibular symptoms.[8] In patients with suspected migraine, the role of possible triggers, such as caffeine, red wine, chocolate, cheese, and fermented foods, should be determined. Some women with migraine have worse symptoms during the perimenstrual cycle or during perimenopause.[11,12]

## Examination and Clinical Testing

Important examinations and clinical tests to perform in a vertiginous patient include the oculomotor examination, an otologic examination, positional testing for BPPV, and a balance/gait examination.

***Ocular examination***
For a thorough physical examination, it is important to begin with an ocular examination including pupillary reactivity and oculomotor movements. The examiner should check smooth pursuit, saccades, and the ability to keep the eyes stable in different positions of gaze. Subtle oculomotor abnormalities can sometimes be the only sign behind a cerebellar dysfunction. A fundoscopic examination can also be helpful to identify oculomotor abnormalities such as ocular torsion. Moreover, in cases of increased intracranial pressure, visual acuity can be normal, and only papilledema may present on fundoscopy. A cover test is also essential to perform to identify any misalignments in the visual axis; of particular concern is any vertical deviation. Vertical skew deviation in the absence of an extraocular muscle abnormality is the vertical misalignment of the eyes that can occur in both acute peripheral lesions and more sinister central disorders, more commonly in the latter. This test is helpful to distinguish between the peripheral or central disorders given peripheral typically causes recover within a week.[13]

***Ear examination***
It is further essential to perform an ear examination. The use of an otoscope can reveal impacted cerumen or any foreign object in the ear canal, removal of which might relieve vertiginous symptoms.[8] Fluid behind the eardrum, perforation, prominent scarring, and other signs of middle ear disease should also be ruled out. A bedside hearing examination can also be performed if the patient complains of hearing impairment, including the Weber and Rinne tests to distinguish between conductive or sensorineural hearing loss.

### Nystagmus

Nystagmus is an involuntary rhythmic oscillatory movement of the eyes. It is essential to examine any nystagmus present in a vertiginous patient. The jerk nystagmus typical of inner ear pathologic condition includes a slow and fast component with the latter used to name the direction of the nystagmus (ie, fast phase to the right is termed right beating nystagmus). It is optimal to use Frenzel glasses that prevent fixation when examining spontaneous nystagmus.

Spontaneous nystagmus is defined as nystagmus present at rest with the eyes in primary position; the head should not be allowed to move. Spontaneous nystagmus can appear in a patient with acute vertigo. In an acute peripheral vestibular loss (eg, vestibular neuritis), spontaneous nystagmus is typically unidirectional and moving in a horizontal and torsional manner, "beating" away from the pathologic ear. When gazing in the direction of the fast phase, the velocity of the nystagmus will increase. The velocity of nystagmus will also reduce with visual fixation. The inability to suppress the nystagmus suggests a central cause.

Nystagmus from a central pathologic condition typically is direction changing depending on gaze position, vertical (upbeat or downbeat), or even purely torsional. However, some central causes for nystagmus can also have features similar to peripheral causes. Gaze-evoked nystagmus occurs with changes in gaze. Caution is warranted if a symmetric horizontal nystagmus occurs with a few beats present in each direction of gaze because this is normal and is called physiologic "endpoint" nystagmus. Asymmetric, prolonged, or more pronounced nystagmus on changing gaze indicates a pathologic condition. Horizontal gaze-evoked nystagmus can occur from use of anticonvulsants, alcohol intoxication, or brainstem or cerebellar disorders.[14]

Headshake nystagmus (HSN) identifies asymmetrical involvement from the vestibular pathways. The examiner shakes the patient's head back and forth vigorously, 20 cycles at the rate of 2 per second (2 Hz). At the end of the head shaking, the eyes are examined for nystagmus with the direction of the fast phase beating toward the healthy ear. This test is best done using Frenzel lenses in order to block visual fixation. Not all patients with unilateral vestibular loss will have a positive HSN test. HSN can also occur in cerebellar dysfunction.[15,16] Those patients with symmetric vestibular involvement will have a negative HSN test.

Positional nystagmus should be checked in every patient that reports dizziness, to rule out BPPV. Nystagmus should be checked in both the Dix-Hallpike maneuver and the roll test, described in detail in later discussion. It is important to first identify any spontaneous nystagmus before proceeding with positional testing in order to avoid the enhanced spontaneous nystagmus that often occurs when placed in different head positions. Enhanced spontaneous nystagmus can cause clinicians to mistakenly diagnose BPPV.

### Dix-Hallpike test

This maneuver is the gold-standard test for diagnosing the most common location for BPPV (the posterior canal) and confirms the displacement of otoconia (calcium carbonate crystals) into the semicircular canals (SCC). It is a quick and easy bedside test that positions the head in a manner for gravity to cause displaced otoconia to move and reproduce the patient symptoms while the examiner looks for nystagmus. The direction of nystagmus along with the vertigo symptom (and sometimes nausea) indicates which SCC is involved (**Table 2**).

To check for posterior canal BPPV, the most common location, the patient sits upright on a flat examination table wearing Frenzel glasses. Throughout the test, the

**Table 2**
**Types of nystagmus with each affected semicircular canals**

| Semicircular Canal | | Type of Nystagmus |
|---|---|---|
| Posterior SCC | Cupulolithiasis | Persistent upbeating nystagmus torsional toward the affected ear |
| | Canalolithiasis | Transient upbeating nystagmus torsional toward the affected ear |
| Horizontal SCC | Cupulolithiasis | Persistent ageotropic |
| | Canalolithiasis | Transient geotropic |
| Superior SCC | Cupulolithiasis | Persistent downbeating nystagmus torsional toward the affected ear |
| | Canalolithiasis | Persistent downbeating nystagmus torsional toward the affected ear |

patient has to keep their eyes open. The examiner moves the patient's head 45° to one side and brings the patient to the supine position with head hyperextended 30° below the horizon (head can be held hanging over the edge of the table). The typical BPPV nystagmus begins after a latent period of a few seconds and then reduces within 1 minute. The test should be performed for each side. Alternatively, examiners can perform this test with the head rotated 45°, but the patient lies on their side with no hyperextension of the neck.[17] It is the side of the head facing the ground that is being tested each time.

### Roll test
A supine roll test should be performed to evaluate horizontal SCC BPPV. The patient is initially supine with head elevated ~30°. Next, the head is rotated 90° to one side while nystagmus and vertigo are assessed. Once the direction of the nystagmus is determined, the head is then returned to the neutral supine position. After any further elicited nystagmus has subsided, the head is then turned 90° to the opposite side, and the eyes are once again observed for nystagmus. In horizontal SCC BPPV, the nystagmus may be described as either geotropic or apogeotropic when in the roll test. Geotropic is horizontal nystagmus beating toward the undermost ear (toward the earth). Ageotropic is horizontal nystagmus beating toward the uppermost ear (away from the earth).

### Head thrust test
The head thrust test (also called the head impulse test) is performed to evaluate the vestibulo-ocular reflex (VOR). The patient is asked to fix their gaze at a near target point (typically the examiners nose about an arm's length away). The head is moved in an unpredictable direction by 10° to 20° with a small-amplitude (5°–15°), high-acceleration (3000°–4000°/s²), and moderate velocity (~200°/s) angular rotation.[18] A normally functioning VOR ensures the eyes remain fixed on the target. However, in vestibular hypofunction, the eyes move with the head rotation, and upon ceasing the head rotation, make a quick refixation saccade to position bring the eyes back to the target. In horizontal SCC hypofunction, the corrective saccades occur when the head is moved toward the lesioned ear. If there is bilateral vestibular hypofunction, the head impulse test may be abnormal on both sides. This test is more sensitive in patients with complete loss of function of the labyrinth of one side as compared with incomplete hypofunction.[19,20]

*Romberg test*
In the Romberg test, the patient is made to stand on a firm surface with feet together and arms folded against the chest. This test is performed first with the eyes open and then closed. Inability to maintain a straight posture or occurrence of sway with both eyes open and closed suggests a pathologic condition, although this test cannot locate where. Abnormal test results may be due to peripheral neuropathy, cerebellar pathologic condition, or vestibular hypofunction among other causes. If the sway is present only with the eyes closed, then the patient may have difficulty using vestibular information. Next, the test is repeated while the patient stands on a 20-cm-thick foam cushion, which alters the proprioceptive input. In bilateral vestibular loss, there is commonly an inability to maintain an upright position standing on foam with eyes closed. The Romberg test is not diagnostic for vestibular hypofunction.

## Vestibular Function Testing

*Electronystagmography/videonystagmography*
Electronystagmography/videonystagmography (ENG/VNG) involves the use of electrodes/video to measure eye motion and examine oculomotor function as well as nystagmus. It is a helpful tool for evaluating vestibular disorders; however, it is more sensitive and specific for central vestibular diseases than peripheral.[9,21]

*Caloric testing*
The caloric test is one component of the ENG/VNG and considered the gold-standard measure of unilateral vestibular hypofunction (UVH). It is the only test that measures each labyrinth separately. Cold and warm water or air is flushed into the external auditory canal leading to creation of a temperature gradient. This gradient causes endolymphatic flow in the horizontal SCC. In addition, the eighth cranial nerve is directly stimulated due to the gradient-induced flow, causing nystagmus (and sometimes nausea). The slow components of the induced nystagmus from each stimulation are compared to identify the side of lesion.

*Rotational chair testing*
Another useful test for vestibular hypofunction is the rotatory chair test, a gold-standard test for bilateral vestibular hypofunction because it measures function from the combined inputs of each labyrinth. The patient is secured to a chair that rotates in different speeds and directions while eye movements are measured. To determine the extent of the pathologic condition, the velocity and position of the resulting eye rotations are compared with the chair rotation. The metrics are also compared with healthy controls. This test can be helpful in measuring vestibular function in pediatric and disabled populations, although it involves expensive equipment.

*Vestibular evoked myogenic potentials testing*
The otolith end organs can be stimulated with sound or bone-conducted vibration, which generates a myogenic potential that can be recorded. It has recently gained significant clinical importance and is now considered a standard test. Two methods are offered: the cervical vestibular-evoked myogenic potentials record surface electromyography (EMG) from the sternocleidomastoid muscles and assess the saccular otolith organ; the ocular vestibular-evoked myogenic potentials version records surface EMG from the inferior oblique extraocular muscle and assesses the utricular otolith organ. Patients with vestibular hypofunction may have absent VEMPs on the side of the lesion.

## PATHOLOGIC CONDITIONS OF THE PERIPHERAL VESTIBULAR SYSTEM
### Unilateral Vestibular Hypofunction

Pathologic conditions that are typically included under the umbrella of UVH include vestibular neuritis, labyrinthitis, unilateral Menieres disease, and perilymphatic fistula.

Vestibular neuritis can be caused by viral, autoimmune causes, or vascular mechanisms. Labyrinthitis can be caused due to bacterial infection of labyrinthine fluids. Both clinically present as an acute onset of imbalance and rotary vertigo, with nausea and a spontaneous horizontal nystagmus. It is diagnosed with a reduced or absence of response in the horizontal SCC when ENG and caloric tests are performed. Hearing loss is present with labyrinthitis, which distinguishes it from vestibular neuritis.

Menieres disease typically presents with an acute episode of hearing impairment, tinnitus, and vertigo lasting for hours. The pathogenesis putatively involves an increase in endolymphatic fluid that causes distention of the membranous tissues. The diagnosis is confirmed using audiogram, ENG (caloric test), or a high-resolution MRI of the inner ear after injecting gadolinium.[15]

### Benign Paroxysmal Positional Vertigo

BPPV is characterized by recurrent episodes of positional vertigo lasting seconds to minutes. The widely accepted theory of pathophysiology creating BPPV is canalithiasis. This mechanism involves otoconia freely floating inside the lumen of the SCC, having become displaced from the utricle. When patients change head position, an atypical stimulation of the SCC results in nystagmus and vertigo in the plane of the affected SCC.[22] The otoconia may attach to the cupula of the affected SCC and cause a persistent positional nystagmus (termed cupulolithiasis). In both types, posterior SCC is most commonly affected ($\sim$75%) followed by horizontal SCC ($\sim$20%). Rarely does BPPV affect the anterior SCC, although multiple SCC BPPV, including bilateral BPPV, can occur.[21,23,24] The types of nystagmus with the affected semicircular canals have been mentioned in **Table 2**.

A diagnosis for posterior canal BPPV is made when vertigo associated with torsional, upbeating nystagmus is provoked by the Dix-Hallpike maneuver. Horizontal canal BPPV is diagnosed with a horizontal nystagmus in the supine roll test.

## THE PHYSICAL THERAPY MANAGEMENT OF VESTIBULAR DISORDERS

There has been moderate to strong evidence that vestibular rehabilitation is an effective and safe modality in UVH and BPPV.[25–27] It has been recorded that patients after resection of an acoustic neuroma recover balance earlier than if not treated.[28] Likewise, patients suffering from acute unilateral vestibular neuritis have shown normalization of postural sway within a significantly shorter time course than those without treatment.[29] Physical therapy has also improved symptoms in patients with vestibular migraine.[30,31] The goal is for patients to develop a home exercise program addressing their limitations while safely improving function and symptoms.

### Unilateral Vestibular Hypofunction

Vestibular exercises are prescribed to treat the gaze and gait instability experienced by patients with vestibular hypofunction. The exercises promote CNS compensation based on repeated exposure to specific stimuli under different conditions. The goals of the therapy include demonstration of improved gaze stability during head movement, decreased sensitivity to motion, improvement in static and dynamic postural stability, and the return to normal activities of daily life. It is essential for patients to be aware of the approximate 6 to 12 weeks of recovery time required, dependent on the extent of hypofunction. Patients benefit most when reinforced about compliance with the exercises.

### Gaze stability exercises

These exercises aim to reduce the instability of gaze during head movement that occurs when the VOR is impaired. This type of exercise exposes the patient to retinal slip, which implies visual images move off the fovea of the retina (during head motion) and cause a blurring of vision. Repeated stimuli of the retinal slip improve the CNS adaptation.[32] Patients are instructed to avoid excessive retinal slip and ensure their focus remains stable on the target during head motion.

Generally, these exercises are progressed in difficulty from sitting to standing and then during ambulation. Difficulty can also be increased by using a distracting background around the target and varying distance from the target. Surface supports can also be adjusted, such as standing on a solid surface, grass, a foam pad, or in sand.

### Postural stability exercises

Most patients suffering from vestibular disorders have balance dysfunction too. The aim of postural stability exercises is to improve balance. Exercises should be safe, within the limitations of the patient's abilities, and challenging to perform as part of a home exercise program. These exercises are generally progressed in terms of difficulty. Some examples include the following:

1. Stand with feet shoulder-width apart, arms across the chest. Progress to bringing feet closer together, then close eyes or stand on foam.
2. Attempt to walk with heel touching toe on a firm surface. Progress to now walk on carpet.
3. Practice walking 5 steps and turning 180° (left and right). Progress to making smaller turns and closing eyes.
4. Walk and move the head side to side, up and down. Progress to counting backward from 100 while doing so.

### Motion sensitivity (habituation) exercises

When continual dizziness symptoms persist, patients may be provided habituation exercises. These exercises reduce the response to a provocative movement by repeating the movement. Over time, the provoking stimuli are less provocative. The clinician must determine the provoking position in order to decide the exercises for the patient. The patient should be guided that symptoms generally reduce within 2 weeks from initiation.

### Benign Paroxysmal Positional Vertigo

The goal of treatment in BPPV is the resolution of nystagmus and associated symptoms, but also includes a rapid return to regular daily activities. New guidelines for the management of BPPV suggest that medications are rarely needed and expensive vestibular function tests are unnecessary.[23] Clinicians should educate patients about the impact of BPPV on their safety and the chances for disease recurrence and emphasize follow-up.

Many different maneuvers exist for the treatment of BPPV. Two treatments are discussed. Before the physical therapy maneuvers for BPPV are performed, the patient should be warned of symptoms during and after the procedures. The patient may feel vertigo, nausea, and disorientation during the maneuvers that can be slightly distressing. After the treatment, sometimes symptoms are reported to subside immediately. In many cases, mild instability and motion sickness might persist for a few hours.

***Canalith repositioning maneuver for treatment of the posterior semicircular canal BPPV (also known as the Epley maneuver)***
The patient is made to sit in an upright position with the head turned 45° toward the affected ear (as diagnosed by Dix-Hallpike test). The patient is then brought to the supine position with head extended 20°. This position is then maintained until the nystagmus and vertigo stops. Next, the head is turned 90° toward the unaffected side (while extension is maintained) and held until the nystagmus and vertigo stop. From here, the patient rolls onto the unaffected side (lateral decubitus) and waits until the nystagmus and vertigo stop. To complete the maneuver, the patient is brought back to the upright sitting position.

***Liberatory/Semont maneuver for treatment of the posterior semicircular canal BPPV***
The patient is made to sit in the sitting upright position with head turned horizontally 45° away from the affected side. The patient is brought quickly to the side lying position of the affected side (lying on the affected ear), and the head will be turned up toward the ceiling. The patient remains in this position for 1 minute. Next, the patient is moved quickly 180° such that the patient is now lying on the unaffected side with the head faced down. This position is held for about 1 minute. The patient is slowly moved back to the sitting upright position.

## VESTIBULAR MIGRAINE

Vestibular migraine is characterized by vestibular symptoms (ie, vertigo, imbalance, nausea) with or without a headache. To make this diagnosis, the patient should have at least 5 episodes with vestibular symptoms of moderate or severe intensity, lasting for 5 minutes to 72 hours and current or previous history of migraine with or without aura according to the International Classification of Headache Disorders.[33] In addition, they should have one or more migraine features in at least 50% of vestibular episodes and other vestibular or migraine causes not accounted for.

Vestibular migraine can be inherited in an autosomal dominant pattern. There are various theories behind the mechanism of this disease, including spreading cortical depression, pathologic channels that affect different neurotransmitters, and vascular anomalies.[34]

In most cases, vestibular migraine is well managed with diet and medication. Uncontrolled migraine can worsen with physical therapy and may be contraindicated for it. Patients with migraine can have significant improvement in functional outcomes after vestibular rehabilitation. However, with vestibular hypofunction also present in the patient, there is often a poor response.

The vestibular rehabilitation in patients with migraine generally follows the principles described above, including BPPV treatments given the 2 to 3 times increased incidence that can occur in vestibular migraine. Vestibular rehabilitation should be attempted when chronic, lingering symptoms of head motion induce dizziness, vertigo, or imbalance. The rehabilitation will not stop the migraine episodes, but can ameliorate the interictal symptoms.

## REFERENCES

1. Neuhauser HK. The epidemiology of dizziness and vertigo. Handb Clin Neurol 2016;137:67–82.
2. Palmeri R, Dulebohn SC. Vertigo, benign paroxysmal position (BPPV). In: StatPearls. Treasure Island (FL): StatPearls Publishing; 2018. Available at: https://www.ncbi.nlm.nih.gov/books/NBK470308/.

3. Kroenke K, Hoffman RM, Einstadter D. How common are various causes of dizziness? A critical review. South Med J 2000;93(2):160–7. Available at: http://www.ncbi.nlm.nih.gov/pubmed/10701780.
4. Hogue JD. Office evaluation of dizziness. Prim Care 2015;42(2):249–58.
5. Kerber K, Callaghan B, Telian S, et al. Dizziness symptom type prevalence and overlap: a US nationally representative survey. Am J Med 2017;130(12):1465.e1-9.
6. Reilly BM. Dizziness. In: Walker HK, Hall WD, Hurst JW, editors. Clinical Methods: The History, Physical, and Laboratory Examinations. 3rd edition. Boston: Butterworths; 1990. Chapter 212. Available at: https://www.ncbi.nlm.nih.gov/books/NBK325/.
7. Zhao J, Piccirillo J, Spitznagel E, et al. Predictive capability of historical data for diagnosis of dizziness. Otol Neurotol 2011;32(2):284–90.
8. Chawla N, Olshaker J. Diagnosis and management of dizziness and vertigo. Med Clin North Am 2006;90(2):291–304.
9. Post RE, Dickerson LM. Dizziness: a diagnostic approach. Am Fam Physician 2010;82(4):361–8.
10. Cohn A. Evaluation and management of the dizzy patient. South Med J 1975;68(5):584–90.
11. Polensek SH, Tusa RJ. Nystagmus during attacks of vestibular migraine: an aid in diagnosis. Audiol Neurootol 2010;15:241–6.
12. Grunfeld E, Gresty MA. Relationship between motion sick- ness, migraine and menstruation in crew members of a 'round the world' yacht race. Brain Res Bull 1998;47:433–6.
13. Mantokoudis G, Schubert M, Saber Tehrani A, et al. Early adaptation and compensation of clinical vestibular responses after unilateral vestibular deafferentation surgery. Otol Neurotol 2014;35(1):148–54.
14. Welgampola MS, Bs MB, Bradshaw AP, et al. Bedside assessment of acute dizziness and vertigo. Neurol Clin 2015;33:551–64.
15. Walther LE. Current diagnostic procedures for diagnosing vertigo and dizziness. GMS Curr Top Otorhinolaryngol Head Neck Surg 2017;16:Doc02.
16. Choi JY, Jung I, Jung JM, et al. Characteristics and mechanism of perverted head-shaking nystagmus in central lesions: video-oculography analysis. Clin Neurophysiol 2016;127(9):2973–8.
17. Cohen H. Side-lying as an alternative to the dix-hallpike test of the posterior canal. Otol Neurotol 2004;25(2):130–4.
18. Halmagyi GM, Curthoys IS. A clinical sign of canal paresis. Arch Neurol 1988;45(7):737–9.
19. Harvey SA, Wood DJ. The oculocephalic response in the evaluation of the dizzy patient. Laryngoscope 1996;106:6–9.
20. Schubert MC, Tusa RJ, Herdman SJ, et al. Optimizing the sensitivity of the head thrust test for identifying vestibular hypofunction. Phys Ther 2004;84:151–8.
21. Hoffman RM, Einstadter D, Kroenke K. Evaluating dizziness. Am J Med 1999;107:468.
22. Schubert MC. Vestibular disorders. In: Herdman SJ, editor. Vestibular rehabilitation. 4th edition. Philadelphia: FA Davis; 2013. Chapter 21. p. 965-95
23. Bhattacharyya N, Gubbels SP, Schwartz SR, et al. Clinical practice guideline: benign paroxysmal positional vertigo (update). Otolaryngol Head Neck Surg 2017;156(3_suppl):S1–47.

24. Cakir B, Ercan I, Cakir Z, et al. What is the true incidence of horizontal semicircular canal benign paroxysmal positional vertigo? Otolaryngol Head Neck Surg 2006;134(3):451–4.
25. Brodovsky J, Vnenchak M. Vestibular rehabilitation for unilateral peripheral vestibular dysfunction. Phys Ther 2013;93(3):293–8.
26. Whitney SL, Alghadir AH, Anwer S. Recent evidence about the effectiveness of vestibular rehabilitation. Curr Treat Options Neurol 2016;18(13):1–15.
27. Alghadir A, Iqbal Z, Whitney S. An update on vestibular physical therapy. J Chin Med Assoc 2013;76(1):1–8.
28. Herdman SJ, Clendaniel RA, Mattox DE, et al. Vestibular adaptation exercises and recovery: acute stage after acoustic neuroma resection. Otolaryngol Head Neck Surg 1995;113:77–87.
29. Strupp M, Arbusow V, Maag KP, et al. Vestibular exer- cises improve central vestibulo-spinal compensation after an acute unilateral peripheral vestibular lesion: a prospec- tive clinical study. Neurology 1998;51:838–44.
30. Sugaya N, Arai M, Goto F. Is the headache in patients with vestibular migraine attenuated by vestibular rehabilitation? Front Neurol 2017;8:1–7.
31. Gottshall KR, Moore RJ, Hoffer ME. Vestibular rehabilitation for migraine-associated dizziness. Int Tinnitus J 2005;11(1):81–4.
32. Schubert MC, Migliaccio A, Clendaniel R, et al. Mechanism of dynamic visual acuity recovery with vestibular rehabilitation. Arch Phys Med Rehabil 2008; 89(3):500–7.
33. Headache Classification Committee of the International Headache Society (IHS). The international classification of headache disorders, 3rd edition (beta version). Cephalalgia 2013;33(9):629–808.
34. Lempert T. Vestibular migraine. Semin Neurol 2013;33:212–8.

# Head and Neck Masses

Kenneth Yan, MD, PhD, Nishant Agrawal, MD, Zhen Gooi, MD*

## KEYWORDS

- Head and neck cancer • Laryngeal cancer • Cutaneous head and neck cancer
- Melanoma • Oral cancer • Nasopharyngeal cancer • Oropharyngeal cancer
- Hypopharyngeal cancer

## KEY POINTS

- Head and neck cancers should be included in the differential diagnosis for a patient with a head and neck mass who presents to the primary care physician. They may present with nonspecific symptoms, including pain, otalgia, dysphagia, and sore throat, or an asymptomatic neck mass.
- Smoking and alcohol use are strongly associated with many types of head and neck malignancies.
- Head and neck cancer is frequently diagnosed with computed tomography or MRI imaging in conjunction with a tissue biopsy. In areas that are difficult to examine, biopsy is often performed in conjunction with endoscopic evaluation in the operating room. Staging is based on size or local invasion, nodal status, and distant metastases.
- Human papillomavirus–associated oropharyngeal cancer represents a unique subtype of head and neck cancers with a different patient population, modified staging criteria, and improved prognosis.
- Early stage head and neck cancers are usually treated with single modality treatment involving either surgery or radiation therapy. Late stage cancers require multimodality treatment involving a combination of surgery, radiation, and chemotherapy with significant patient morbidity.

## INTRODUCTION

Head and neck cancers account for 4% of all cancers in the United States each year.[1] It is expected that there will be more than 64,000 new cases of head and neck cancer diagnosed in 2018 in the United States, and nearly 11,000 deaths.[1] A significant proportion of these cancers are discovered incidentally in the form of painless neck masses by primary care physicians or dentists, and patients may also present with

Disclosure Statement: There are no commercial or financial conflicts of interest or funding sources.

Section of Otolaryngology, Department of Surgery, University of Chicago Medicine, Chicago, IL, USA

* Corresponding author. The University of Chicago Medicine and Biological Sciences, 5841 South Maryland Avenue, Room E-103, MC1035, Chicago, IL 60637.

E-mail address: zgooi@surgery.bsd.uchicago.edu

Med Clin N Am 102 (2018) 1013–1025

https://doi.org/10.1016/j.mcna.2018.06.012

nonspecific symptoms of dysphonia, dysphagia, and otalgia. It is essential for the internist to have a basic idea of the workup of common head and neck cancers that could present in the office. The purpose of this review is to provide a basic background on head and neck cancers in order to recognize presenting symptoms and facilitate appropriate workup.

## CUTANEOUS MALIGNANCIES

Both melanoma and nonmelanoma skin cancers frequently occur in the head and neck region. Nonmelanoma skin cancers are the most common malignancies in the United States. The total number of nonmelanoma skin cancers in the United States was estimated to be more than 5.4 million in 2012, and this number has been steadily increasing over time.[2,3] Around 70% to 80% of skin cancers are basal cell carcinomas (BCC); 15% are squamous cell cancers (SCC), and less than 5% are melanomas.[4] There is a well-established relationship between UV-B radiation and the development of cutaneous malignancies, particularly SCC.[5]

### Clinical Presentation

Any new, enlarging, or ulcerative skin lesions warrant further investigation for cutaneous malignancy. BCC can be divided into several major clinical subtypes: nodular, superficial multicentric, pigmented, morpheaform, and fibroepithelioma.[6,7] Cutaneous squamous cell carcinoma usually presents as an indurated and often scaly papule, plaque, or nodule.[7] Actinic keratoses are extremely common lesions that form as a result of sun exposure and are thought to be premalignant lesions that may progress to SCC. These lesions are often difficult to distinguish from SCC.[8]

Lesions suspicious for melanoma are classically identified using ABCDE criteria (asymmetry, border irregularity, color variegation, diameter >6 mm, evolving).[9] Melanomas can also present on mucosal membranes such as within the oral or nasal cavity; half of mucosal melanomas are in the head and neck region.[10] These melanomas tend to have late presentations and poor prognoses.

### Diagnosis

A tissue biopsy should be performed to confirm the diagnosis of cutaneous head and neck cancer. A shave biopsy is used to obtain superficial cells from a suspicious lesion for pathology but will not provide information about depth of invasion. A punch biopsy or excisional biopsy will provide additional information about the thickness or depth of a lesion. Melanoma thickness, called the Breslow thickness, is strongly related to patient prognosis. Therefore, a punch or excisional biopsy is the preferred option.

All cutaneous malignancies of the head and neck are staged using the American Joint Committee on Cancer (AJCC) TNM staging system. T staging for BCC and SCC depends on size, invasion of adjacent structures, and high-risk features.[11] High-risk features include depth of invasion, perineural invasion, poor differentiation, and primary tumor sites of the non-hair-bearing lip and ear.

Nodal designation (N) is an assessment of regional lymph node metastases. A full discussion on N staging for head and neck cancers are reviewed in the later discussion of oral cancer. Metastasis (M) designation depends on whether the tumor has distant metastases. BCC is rarely metastatic, whereas cutaneous SCC has a 5% rate of regional neck metastases.[4,12] Overall tumor stage depends on TNM designation: a T1N0M0 cancer is stage I; a T2N0M0 cancer is stage II; a T3 or N1 cancer is stage III; and T4 or N2 status is stage IV.

Melanoma is also staged using the TNM staging system. The key difference between the staging of melanoma compared with nonmelanoma cutaneous malignancies is that melanoma T staging depends largely on the Breslow thickness as described earlier and the presence or absence of ulcerations.[13] This highlights the importance of melanoma thickness in determining patient prognosis.

### Treatment

There are numerous treatment modalities for nonmelanoma cutaneous malignancies, but the mainstay of treatment is surgery. For head and neck BCC and SCC, lesions can be divided into low- and high-risk categories based on size, location, borders, patient immunosuppression, or previous radiation, as well as specific features on pathology.[14] Low-risk lesions can be treated with curettage and electrodessication or surgical excision with 4-mm margins. For high-risk lesions, Moh's micrographic surgery is a good option with a 1.4% 5-year recurrence rate for primary BCC and a 3.9% 5-year recurrence rate for primary SCC.[15,16] Wide local excision with circumferential margin analysis is another option.[4] A neck dissection (removal of lymph nodes in the neck) is indicated for clinical or radiographic disease in the neck. Radiation is reserved for positive nodal disease, positive surgical margins, or poor surgical candidates.

Melanomas are also treated with surgical excision with adequate margins. A margin of 1 cm is necessary for lesions up to 1 mm in thickness.[17] A margin of 2 cm is required for lesions greater than 2 mm in thickness.[18] A sentinel lymph node biopsy is a procedure whereby a radiolabel is injected at the melanoma site and the sentinel lymph nodes, the primary lymph nodes that take up dye, are excised to assess for tumor. Sentinel lymph node biopsy has been proven to be effective for intermediate thickness and thick melanomas and is standard practice today.[19] Thin melanomas (a thickness of <0.75 mm) have good prognosis and can often be treated with surgical excision alone. Melanomas with positive sentinel lymph nodes warrant consideration of completion nodal dissection, radiotherapy, or chemotherapy.

### ORAL CAVITY CANCER

The oral cavity can be divided into several anatomic subsites: the lips, the buccal mucosa or the mucosa lining the inside of the cheek, the alveolar ridges along the upper and lower dentition, the hard palate, the floor of the mouth, the oral tongue, and the retromolar trigone, which is located posterior to the second mandibular molar. There are expected to be more than 30,000 new cases of oral cavity cancer in the United States in 2018.[1]

There is a cumulative effect for smoking and alcohol use in the risk of oral cavity cancer.[20] Also of note, betel quid chewing predisposes patients to buccal mucosa cancer; it has been responsible for a recent increase in oral cavity cancer in Taiwan and other Asian countries.[21] The most common pathologic condition is SCC, accounting for nearly 90% of oral cavity cancers, followed by adenocarcinoma.[22] In addition, other pathologic conditions, such as minor salivary gland cancer and mucosal melanoma, can present in the oral cavity. More than 50% of oral cavity cancers originate in either the tongue or the floor of the mouth.[22]

### Clinical Presentation

Oral cavity cancer frequently presents as an oral mass or nonhealing ulcer, or it can manifest as oral cavity swelling or a whitish or reddish patch within the oral cavity. A white patch is called leukoplakia and a red patch is called erythroplakia; of the 2 presentations, erythroplakia carries the higher cancer risk.[23] Pain is also a common manifestation and tends to worsen with tumor stage.[24] Functional issues, such as dysphagia or involvement of head and neck cranial nerves, are also harbingers of more advanced disease.

Oral cavity cancer metastasizes to the cervical lymph nodes in the neck and can also occasionally present as a painless cervical neck mass.[22] Any patient who presents to the primary care physician with a suspicious oral lesion should be assessed for neck metastases by physical examination. Of note, the submandibular glands are bilateral symmetric palpable masses located inferior to the body of the mandible and are not neck metastases.

### Diagnosis

A biopsy should be performed for any suspicious oral lesion and can usually be performed in an office setting. A computed tomographic (CT) scan with contrast has high sensitivity and specificity for detection of neck metastases and is generally the imaging study of choice.[25] The most common distant metastatic site for oral cavity cancer is the lung,[26] so a CT scan of the chest is performed if clinically indicated in patients with a known smoking history. For advanced stage disease, further imaging PET/CT should also be considered.[27]

Oral cavity cancer is staged by the AJCC TNM staging system. For oral cavity cancers, T designation depends on tumor size, depth of invasion, and invasion of adjacent structures, such as the mandible or maxilla. N designation is an assessment of lymph node status. In older staging criteria, a tumor with a single ipsilateral lymph node 3 cm or less in diameter was designated as N1; tumors with lymph nodes between 3 cm and 6 cm in diameter, or multiple, bilateral, or contralateral lymph nodes were designated as N2; and lymph nodes greater than 6 cm in diameter were characterized as N3.[11] In the eighth edition of the AJCC Cancer Staging Manual, the criteria of extranodal extension, tumor growth outside of the lymph node capsule, were added to N staging of all head and neck cancers.[28] M designation refers to metastatic disease.

### Treatment

Early stage oral cavity cancer is treated by either primary resection or radiation therapy alone.[22] Surgical resection is the mainstay for early stage oral cavity cancer, and radiation is reserved for patients who are poor surgical candidates. Following surgery, reconstruction of the defect with a local, regional, or free flap might be indicated. A neck dissection is performed to address either occult or clinically apparent regional metastasis to the neck. A neck dissection involves removal of lymph nodes at risk of metastasis. The neck dissection aims to preserve anatomic structures, including the internal jugular vein, spinal accessory nerve, and sternocleidomastoid muscle, to avoid treatment morbidity.

Adjuvant radiation or chemoradiation therapy is indicated for high-risk features, such as positive margins, vascular invasion, perineural invasion, extranodal extension, and T3 or T4 tumors.[29] A total dose of 60 to 66 Gy of radiation is given over the course of 6 weeks. When chemotherapy is given as well, single-agent cisplatin is recommended.[30]

## NASOPHARYNGEAL CANCER

Nasopharyngeal cancer (NPC) is a rare malignancy with an overall incidence of less than 1 per 100,000 worldwide.[31] However, the incidence of NPC has a geographic variation with an increased rate of NPC in the Cantonese-speaking population of the Guangdong province of Southern China, Taiwanese and other southern Chinese populations, Southeast Asians, and Alaskan Inuits.[31] This increased rate is related to consumption of preserved foods and nitrosamine-containing fish at a young age, which are also thought to contain Epstein-Barr virus (EBV) activating substances.[31] EBV DNA is frequently isolated from NPCs in these endemic areas.[32,33] Other risk factors for NPC include smoking and occupational formaldehyde exposure.[34] All NPCs are either squamous cell carcinomas or undifferentiated carcinomas.[35] The World Health Organization classifies NPCs into type I–III, where type I NPCs are typical keratinizing squamous cell carcinoma and type III NPCs are undifferentiated. Of note, type III NPC accounts for greater than 95% of cancers in high-incidence areas.[36]

### Clinical Presentation

Nasopharyngeal carcinoma presents at a late stage because of the nonspecific nature of presenting symptoms.[35] In retrospective analyses, the most common presenting symptom in patients was a neck mass from a cervical metastasis.[37] Patients with NPC may also present with nasal symptoms, such as nasal discharge, bleeding, or obstruction, and ear symptoms, such as aural fullness or a unilateral effusion from Eustachian tube obstruction.[37] As such, any adult patient who presents to the primary care physician with unexplained unilateral hearing loss or middle ear effusion will need to be referred to an otolaryngologist to rule out NPC.

### Diagnosis

All patients with suspected nasopharyngeal carcinoma should undergo endoscopic evaluation with a biopsy of the tumor as well as imaging. In general, CT is excellent at determining soft tissue extension in the nasopharynx, bony invasion, and parapharyngeal spread. However, MRI is the preferred modality in determining skull base involvement.[38]

NPC is staged using the AJCC TNM staging system. In NPC, T staging is solely based on degree of invasion into adjacent anatomic structures rather than size.[28] The N designation for NPC differs from that of other head and neck cancers: in short, unilateral metastases are classified as N1; bilateral metastases are classified as N2; and metastases larger than 6 cm in diameter or those that present in the supraclavicular fossa are classified as N3.[28]

### Treatment

NPC is sensitive to radiation therapy and technically challenging to resect operatively. Therefore, chemoradiation therapy is the mainstay of treatment.[35] Adjuvant chemotherapy is also used in advanced stage disease involving administration of either cisplatin or carboplatin along with 5-fluorouracil.[39,40]

## OROPHARYNGEAL CANCER

The oropharynx has 4 subsites: the base of the tongue, tonsils, soft palate, and pharyngeal wall. Historically, primary risk factors for oropharyngeal cancer were smoking and alcohol use.[41] Over the past 2 decades, however, the human papillomavirus (HPV) has been recognized as an etiologic agent for most oropharyngeal cancers within the United States and Europe.[42] HPV-related oropharyngeal tumors are discussed later in this text.

### Clinical Presentation

The most common subsites of oropharyngeal cancer are the tonsils, followed by the base of the tongue.[43] The oropharynx should be visualized in any patient presenting with symptoms of a persistent sore throat, odynophagia, otalgia, dysphagia, or globus sensation. In addition, oropharyngeal cancer frequently presents as an otherwise asymptomatic cervical neck mass, especially in middle-aged patients with HPV-associated cancers.[43]

### Diagnosis

Imaging studies involving either CT or MRI of the neck should be performed in any patient with suspected oropharyngeal cancer. Dedicated chest imaging should be considered in addition to PET/CT for patients with advanced stage disease. In addition, all patients with a new diagnosis of oropharyngeal cancer should undergo a thorough endoscopic evaluation with a biopsy of the suspected primary site. The rate of synchronous second primaries in patients with oropharyngeal cancer has been found to be around 10%, with an increased incidence in smokers.[44]

The staging of oropharyngeal cancers is based on AJCC TNM designation and differs for HPV-associated and HPV-negative cancers.[28] For HPV-negative cancers, T designation depends on tumor size and invasion of adjacent structures. N designation is similar to oral cavity cancer and depends on lymph node size, location, and extranodal extension. M designation depends on distant metastases. The overall stage is based on TNM designation and is described earlier in this text.

### Treatment

In general, early stage oropharyngeal cancer is treated with single- modality treatment: either surgery or primary radiation therapy.[45] The recent development of transoral robotic surgeries has provided the significant advantage of improved exposure and manipulation of the tumor site to facilitate excision of oropharyngeal cancers with decreased patient morbidity as compared with traditional approaches involving mandibulectomy and pharyngotomies for tumor access.[46] The decision for adjuvant therapy following surgical resection with either radiation or chemoradiation therapy is dictated by the presence of adverse features, such as extracapsular nodal spread, positive margins, T3 or T4 primary, N2 or N3 nodal disease, or perineural invasion.

Patients with later stage cancers are treated with multimodality therapy. Options include concurrent chemoradiation therapy versus surgery followed by radiation or chemoradiation therapy. Large randomized controlled trials have shown a benefit for chemoradiation compared with radiation therapy alone for patients with extracapsular nodal extension or positive margins.[47–52]

## HUMAN PAPILLOMAVIRUS–RELATED CANCERS

Oropharyngeal squamous cell carcinoma has increased in incidence since the 1970s, specifically among young, Caucasian, nonsmoking men.[53] This increase is from changing sexual behaviors and the role of HPV in oropharyngeal SCC involving the tongue base or tonsil.[54,55] The high-risk HPV subtypes 16 and 18 are the most common etiologic agents for oropharyngeal cancer and are thought to exert their oncogenic effects by binding and degrading p53 and retinoblastoma tumor suppressor via E6 and E7 viral oncoproteins.[56]

### Prevention and Testing

HPV is well publicized as the leading cause of cervical cancer worldwide.[57] However, unlike cervical cancer, there is no recognized premalignant state for HPV-related oropharyngeal cancer. Therefore, there have been no validated screening protocols for early detection of these cancers. In the United States, there are 2 HPV vaccines that are currently available for use. The quadrivalent vaccine, Gardasil, protects against infection with HPV-6, -11, -16, and -18.[58] It is licensed for use in girls and women and boys and men between the ages of 9 and 26. This vaccine has been shown to effectively prevent cervical and anal cancers as well as cervical warts. The bivalent vaccine, Cervarix, protects against HPV-16 and -18 and is licensed for use for prevention of cervical cancer.[59]

### Treatment Considerations

HPV positivity is an independent positive prognostic indicator of patient survival in oropharyngeal cancer.[60] HPV-positive cancers are exquisitely sensitive to radiation therapy,[61] and in large clinical trials of patients with oropharyngeal cancer treated with chemoradiation therapy, HPV-positive patients have improved responses and prognoses.[60,62] Because of this difference, oropharyngeal SCC is recognized as a separate disease entity compared with other pharyngeal head and neck cancers. There is interest in developing treatment deintensification protocols to reduce treatment morbidity for this group of cancers.

## HYPOPHARYNGEAL CARCINOMA

The hypopharynx is bordered by the hyoid bone superiorly and extends inferiorly to the level of the cricoid cartilage. It is divided into 3 subsites: the pyriform sinuses, the postcricoid area, and the posterior pharyngeal wall. Hypopharyngeal cancers account for approximately 4% of head and neck cancers in the United States.[63] There is a strong association between smoking and alcohol use and the development of hypopharyngeal cancer.[20]

### Clinical Presentation

As with NPCs, more than half of hypopharyngeal cancers present at later stages due to the nonspecific nature of symptoms. The most common presenting symptoms are dysphagia, hoarseness, and neck mass.[64]

### Diagnosis

Similar to oropharyngeal tumors, hypopharyngeal cancers are commonly identified on flexible fiber-optic scope examination, and biopsy for histopathological confirmation is obtained in the operating room. Further imaging is performed to identify extent of invasion and regional or distant metastases. MRI is more sensitive but less specific than CT in assessing for cartilaginous invasion.[65] Staging of hypopharyngeal cancer is once again determined by AJCC TNM staging criteria.[28]

### Treatment

Treatment paradigms for hypopharyngeal cancer are similar to that of oropharyngeal cancer. Because most hypopharyngeal cancers are identified at late stage, multimodality therapy is the norm. Both surgery with postoperative radiation and concurrent chemoradiation therapy are treatment options for late stage hypopharyngeal cancer.[66] However, surgical treatment of advanced stage hypopharyngeal cancer usually entails total laryngectomy. Because of the fundamental role of the larynx in speech production in everyday life, total laryngectomy has significant effects on patient quality of life.[67,68] Therefore, most therapies involve concurrent chemoradiation with surgery reserved for salvage therapy.[47–51]

## LARYNGEAL CANCERS

The larynx is a combination of cartilaginous and mucosal structures in the neck that performs 3 key functions of airway protection, respiration, and phonation. It is divided into 3 main regions: the supraglottis, glottis, and subglottis. The supraglottis is further subdivided into the suprahyoid and infrahyoid epiglottis, the arytenoid cartilages, the aryepiglottic folds, and the false vocal cords. The glottis is composed of the true vocal cords and anterior and posterior commissures. The subglottis begins 1 cm below the ventricle to the cricoid and is not divided into further subsites.

Laryngeal cancer is the second most common respiratory cancer and more than 13,000 new cases of laryngeal cancer are expected to be diagnosed in the United States this year.[1] Laryngeal cancer is related to smoking and alcohol use, with a strong dose-dependent effect of smoking.[69] HPV-16 is not related to laryngeal cancer.[70]

### Clinical Presentation

Glottic cancer is the most common laryngeal cancer, followed by supraglottic cancer. Subglottic cancer is very rare.[71] Primary symptoms of supraglottic cancer include dysphagia, odynophagia, and referred otalgia. The patient may present with a palpable neck mass. Glottic tumors tend to be diagnosed early because a glottic mass will manifest as hoarseness.[71] The embryologic origins of the glottis and supraglottis are separate, and because of this, glottic cancers rarely have any associated cervical lymphadenopathy, whereas supraglottic cancers tend to have lymphadenopathy on presentation. Subglottic tumors often present in an emergent setting with airway obstruction.

### Diagnosis

A patient presenting with suspicious symptoms requires fiber-optic scope examination and directed biopsies in the operating room. Clinical examination alone frequently fails to identify the deeper extent of tumor invasion of the laryngeal cartilages, and staging accuracy is significantly increased following endoscopy and imaging.[65] MRI is more sensitive but less specific than CT in assessing for cartilaginous invasion.[65] The rate of synchronous primaries in laryngeal cancer is upwards of 11% and is often lung primaries provided the high association of laryngeal cancer with smoking.[72] Therefore, guidelines recommend chest imaging especially in patients with prior smoking history.

Staging for laryngeal cancer is based on AJCC TNM guidelines. T designation for laryngeal cancer depends on whether the tumor has invaded into adjacent structures and whether the vocal cords are moving normally.[71] N and M designations and overall tumor stages based on TNM designation are similar to that of other head and neck cancers, as discussed previously.

### Treatment

The goal of laryngeal cancer treatment should be laryngeal preservation if possible. For early stage tumors, laryngeal preservation surgery involving partial laryngectomy through either open neck surgery or endoscopic approaches or radiation therapy may be used.[73] Late stage tumors are treated with organ-preservation surgery or concurrent chemoradiation.[73] Neck dissection is performed to address nodal basins at risk for all laryngeal cancers except in the case of early stage glottic tumors, where the propensity of occult nodal metastatic spread is low.

## BENIGN HEAD AND NECK MASSES

The differential diagnosis for a new head and neck mass that presents to the internist's office is extremely broad. For a neck mass in a young patient with concurrent infectious symptoms, infectious causes should be on the top of the differential diagnosis.[74,75] Autoimmune and other rheumatologic diseases can also present as head and neck masses.[76,77] In young patients, congenital neck masses, such as branchial cleft cysts, dermoid cysts, and thyroglossal duct cysts, should be considered in the differential diagnosis.[78] A thyroglossal duct cyst presents as a midline neck mass that may become inflamed or superinfected. Because of its association with the hyoid bone, it frequently will elevate with swallow or protrusion of the tongue. A branchial cleft abnormality can present as a neck mass in a young patient and can be associated with a fistula or sinus tract. A laryngocele or saccular cyst can present as a laryngeal or neck mass and cause similar symptoms as a laryngeal tumor.[79]

A history of neck trauma or surgery should be inquired of any patient with a new head and neck mass. A mucocele is a cystic fluid collection caused by the trapping of mucus from a major or minor salivary gland or a paranasal sinus and frequently forms secondary to trauma.[80] A plunging ranula is a type of mucocele associated with the sublingual gland that will present as a bluish mass on the floor of the mouth. In addition, vascular malformations and vascular tumors such as paragangliomas are included in the differential diagnosis. Neuronal tumors, such as schwannomas, can rarely present in association with any cranial nerve, and manifest as a neck mass. It is important for the internist to obtain a prudent history and physical examination to help narrow the diagnostic possibilities.

## SUMMARY

Although the differential diagnosis for a new head and neck mass is broad, new head and neck cancer should always be a consideration in an adult patient presenting with symptoms of hoarseness, a nagging sore throat, ear pain, or a painless neck mass. There should be a low threshold for referral of these patients to an otolaryngologist for better visualization of laryngeal and pharyngeal structures. When diagnosed early, many head and neck cancers can be treated with surgical excision or radiation therapy with curative intent. A delay in diagnosis will allow tumor growth, infiltration into adjacent tissues, and metastatic spread, which can necessitate more morbid treatments with larger impact on quality of life.

## REFERENCES

1. American Cancer Society, Cancer Facts and Figures 2018. Available at: https://www.cancer.org/research/cancer-facts-statistics.
2. Rogers HW, Weinstock MA, Feldman SR, et al. Incidence Estimate of Nonmelanoma Skin Cancer (Keratinocyte Carcinomas) in the U.S. Population, 2012. JAMA Dermatol 2015;151(10):1081–6.
3. Muzic JG, Schmitt AR, Wright AC, et al. Incidence and trends of basal cell carcinoma and cutaneous squamous cell carcinoma: a population-based study in Olmsted County, Minnesota, 2000 to 2010. Mayo Clin Proc 2017;92(6):890–8.
4. Mydlarz WK, Weber RS, Kupferman ME. Cutaneous malignancy of the head and neck. Surg Oncol Clin N Am 2015;24(3):593–613.
5. Ziegler A, Jonason AS, Leffell DJ, et al. Sunburn and p53 in the onset of skin cancer. Nature 1994;372(6508):773–6.
6. Betti R, Inselvini E, Carducci M, et al. Age and site prevalence of histologic subtypes of basal cell carcinomas. Int J Dermatol 1995;34(3):174–6.
7. Dubas LE, Ingraffea A. Nonmelanoma skin cancer. Facial Plast Surg Clin North Am 2013;21(1):43–53.

8. Salasche SJ. Epidemiology of actinic keratoses and squamous cell carcinoma. J Am Acad Dermatol 2000;42(1 Pt 2):4–7.

9. Abbasi NR, Shaw HM, Rigel DS, et al. Early diagnosis of cutaneous melanoma: revisiting the ABCD criteria. JAMA 2004;292(22):2771–6.

10. Chang AE, Karnell LH, Menck HR. The National Cancer Data Base report on cutaneous and noncutaneous melanoma: a summary of 84,836 cases from the past decade. The American College of Surgeons Commission on Cancer and the American Cancer Society. Cancer 1998;83(8):1664–78.

11. Warner CL, Cockerell CJ. The new seventh edition American Joint Committee on Cancer staging of cutaneous non-melanoma skin cancer: a critical review. Am J Clin Dermatol 2011;12(3):147–54.

12. von Domarus H, Stevens PJ. Metastatic basal cell carcinoma. Report of five cases and review of 170 cases in the literature. J Am Acad Dermatol 1984; 10(6):1043–60.

13. Balch CM, Gershenwald JE, Soong SJ, et al. Final version of 2009 AJCC melanoma staging and classification. J Clin Oncol 2009;27(36):6199–206.

14. Connolly SM, Baker DR, Coldiron BM, et al. AAD/ACMS/ASDSA/ASMS 2012 appropriate use criteria for Mohs micrographic surgery: a report of the American Academy of Dermatology, American College of Mohs Surgery, American Society for Dermatologic Surgery Association, and the American Society for Mohs Surgery. J Am Acad Dermatol 2012;67(4):531–50.

15. Leibovitch I, Huilgol SC, Selva D, et al. Basal cell carcinoma treated with Mohs surgery in Australia II. Outcome at 5-year follow-up. J Am Acad Dermatol 2005;53(3):452–7.

16. Leibovitch I, Huilgol SC, Selva D, et al. Cutaneous squamous cell carcinoma treated with Mohs micrographic surgery in Australia I. Experience over 10 years. J Am Acad Dermatol 2005;53(2):253–60.

17. Veronesi U, Cascinelli N, Adamus J, et al. Thin stage I primary cutaneous malignant melanoma. Comparison of excision with margins of 1 or 3 cm. N Engl J Med 1988;318(18):1159–62.

18. Gillgren P, Drzewiecki KT, Niin M, et al. 2-cm versus 4-cm surgical excision margins for primary cutaneous melanoma thicker than 2 mm: a randomised, multi-centre trial. Lancet 2011;378(9803):1635–42.

19. Morton DL, Thompson JF, Cochran AJ, et al. Final trial report of sentinel-node biopsy versus nodal observation in melanoma. N Engl J Med 2014;370(7):599–609.

20. Hashibe M, Brennan P, Chuang SC, et al. Interaction between tobacco and alcohol use and the risk of head and neck cancer: pooled analysis in the International Head and Neck Cancer Epidemiology Consortium. Cancer Epidemiol Biomarkers Prev 2009;18(2):541–50.

21. Su CC, Yang HF, Huang SJ, et al. Distinctive features of oral cancer in Changhua County: high incidence, buccal mucosa preponderance, and a close relation to betel quid chewing habit. J Formos Med Assoc 2007;106(3):225–33.

22. Funk GF, Karnell LH, Robinson RA, et al. Presentation, treatment, and outcome of oral cavity cancer: a National Cancer Data Base report. Head Neck 2002;24(2):165–80.

23. Jainkittivong A, Swasdison S, Thangpisityotin M, et al. Oral squamous cell carcinoma: a clinicopathological study of 342 Thai cases. J Contemp Dent Pract 2009; 10(5):E033–40.

24. Bagan J, Sarrion G, Jimenez Y. Oral cancer: clinical features. Oral Oncol 2010; 46(6):414–7.

25. Curtin HD, Ishwaran H, Mancuso AA, et al. Comparison of CT and MR imaging in staging of neck metastases. Radiology 1998;207(1):123–30.
26. Liao CT, Wang HM, Chang JT, et al. Analysis of risk factors for distant metastases in squamous cell carcinoma of the oral cavity. Cancer 2007;110(7):1501–8.
27. Fleming AJ Jr, Smith SP Jr, Paul CM, et al. Impact of [18F]-2-fluorodeoxyglucose-positron emission tomography/computed tomography on previously untreated head and neck cancer patients. Laryngoscope 2007;117(7):1173–9.
28. Lydiatt WM, Patel SG, O'Sullivan B, et al. Head and Neck cancers-major changes in the American Joint Committee on cancer eighth edition cancer staging manual. CA Cancer J Clin 2017;67(2):122–37.
29. Hinerman RW, Mendenhall WM, Morris CG, et al. Postoperative irradiation for squamous cell carcinoma of the oral cavity: 35-year experience. Head Neck 2004;26(11):984–94.
30. Bernier J, Domenge C, Ozsahin M, et al. Postoperative irradiation with or without concomitant chemotherapy for locally advanced head and neck cancer. N Engl J Med 2004;350(19):1945–52.
31. Yu MC, Yuan JM. Epidemiology of nasopharyngeal carcinoma. Semin Cancer Biol 2002;12(6):421–9.
32. Gooi Z, Fakhry C, Goldenberg D, et al. AHNS series: do you know your guide-lines?Principles of radiation therapy for head and neck cancer: a review of the National Comprehensive Cancer Network guidelines. Head Neck 2016;38(7): 987–92.
33. Raab-Traub N. Epstein-Barr virus in the pathogenesis of NPC. Semin Cancer Biol 2002;12(6):431–41.
34. Roush GC, Walrath J, Stayner LT, et al. Nasopharyngeal cancer, sinonasal cancer, and occupations related to formaldehyde: a case-control study. J Natl Cancer Inst 1987;79(6):1221–4.
35. Wei WI, Sham JS. Nasopharyngeal carcinoma. Lancet 2005;365(9476):2041–54.
36. Gooi Z, Richmon J, Agrawal N, et al. AHNS Series - Do you know your guidelines? Principles of treatment for nasopharyngeal cancer: a review of the National Comprehensive Cancer Network guidelines. Head Neck 2017;39(2):201–5.
37. Lee AW, Foo W, Law SC, et al. Nasopharyngeal carcinoma: presenting symptoms and duration before diagnosis. Hong Kong Med J 1997;3(4):355–61.
38. Chong VF, Fan YF. Skull base erosion in nasopharyngeal carcinoma: detection by CT and MRI. Clin Radiol 1996;51(9):625–31.
39. Chan AT, Leung SF, Ngan RK, et al. Overall survival after concurrent cisplatin-radiotherapy compared with radiotherapy alone in locoregionally advanced naso-pharyngeal carcinoma. J Natl Cancer Inst 2005;97(7):536–9.
40. Dechaphunkul T, Pruegsanusak K, Sangthawan D, et al. Concurrent chemoradio-therapy with carboplatin followed by carboplatin and 5-fluorouracil in locally advanced nasopharyngeal carcinoma. Head Neck Oncol 2011;3:30.
41. Mashberg A, Boffetta P, Winkelman R, et al. Tobacco smoking, alcohol drinking, and cancer of the oral cavity and oropharynx among U.S. veterans. Cancer 1993; 72(4):1369–75.
42. Chaturvedi AK, Engels EA, Pfeiffer RM, et al. Human papillomavirus and rising oropharyngeal cancer incidence in the United States. J Clin Oncol 2011; 29(32):4294–301.
43. McIlwain WR, Sood AJ, Nguyen SA, et al. Initial symptoms in patients with HPV-positive and HPV-negative oropharyngeal cancer. JAMA Otolaryngol Head Neck Surg 2014;140(5):441–7.

44. Rodriguez-Bruno K, Ali MJ, Wang SJ. Role of panendoscopy to identify synchronous second primary malignancies in patients with oral cavity and oropharyngeal squamous cell carcinoma. Head Neck 2011;33(7):949–53.

45. Selek U, Garden AS, Morrison WH, et al. Radiation therapy for early-stage carcinoma of the oropharynx. Int J Radiat Oncol Biol Phys 2004;59(3):743–51.

46. Moore EJ, Olsen KD, Kasperbauer JL. Transoral robotic surgery for oropharyngeal squamous cell carcinoma: a prospective study of feasibility and functional outcomes. Laryngoscope 2009;119(11):2156–64.

47. Adelstein DJ, Saxton JP, Lavertu P, et al. A phase III randomized trial comparing concurrent chemotherapy and radiotherapy with radiotherapy alone in resectable stage III and IV squamous cell head and neck cancer: preliminary results. Head Neck 1997;19(7):567–75.

48. Brizel DM, Albers ME, Fisher SR, et al. Hyperfractionated irradiation with or without concurrent chemotherapy for locally advanced head and neck cancer. N Engl J Med 1998;338(25):1798–804.

49. Wendt TG, Grabenbauer GG, Rodel CM, et al. Simultaneous radiochemotherapy versus radiotherapy alone in advanced head and neck cancer: a randomized multicenter study. J Clin Oncol 1998;16(4):1318–24.

50. Fu KK, Pajak TF, Trotti A, et al. A Radiation Therapy Oncology Group (RTOG) phase III randomized study to compare hyperfractionation and two variants of accelerated fractionation to standard fractionation radiotherapy for head and neck squamous cell carcinomas: first report of RTOG 9003. Int J Radiat Oncol Biol Phys 2000;48(1):7–16.

51. Ezra P, Noel G, Mazeron JJ. [Randomized trial of radiation therapy versus concomitant chemotherapy and radiation therapy for advanced-stage oropharynx carcinoma]. Cancer Radiother 2000;4(4):324–5 [in French].

52. Calais G, Alfonsi M, Bardet E, et al. Randomized trial of radiation therapy versus concomitant chemotherapy and radiation therapy for advanced-stage oropharynx carcinoma. J Natl Cancer Inst 1999;91(24):2081–6.

53. Canto MT, Devesa SS. Oral cavity and pharynx cancer incidence rates in the United States, 1975-1998. Oral Oncol 2002;38(6):610–7.

54. Gillison ML, Koch WM, Capone RB, et al. Evidence for a causal association between human papillomavirus and a subset of head and neck cancers. J Natl Cancer Inst 2000;92(9):709–20.

55. Chaturvedi AK, Engels EA, Anderson WF, et al. Incidence trends for human papillomavirus-related and -unrelated oral squamous cell carcinomas in the United States. J Clin Oncol 2008;26(4):612–9.

56. Rampias T, Sasaki C, Weinberger P, et al. E6 and e7 gene silencing and transformed phenotype of human papillomavirus 16-positive oropharyngeal cancer cells. J Natl Cancer Inst 2009;101(6):412–23.

57. Walboomers JM, Jacobs MV, Manos MM, et al. Human papillomavirus is a necessary cause of invasive cervical cancer worldwide. J Pathol 1999;189(1):12–9.

58. D'Souza G, Dempsey A. The role of HPV in head and neck cancer and review of the HPV vaccine. Prev Med 2011;53(Suppl 1):S5–11.

59. Harper DM, Franco EL, Wheeler CM, et al. Sustained efficacy up to 4.5 years of a bivalent L1 virus-like particle vaccine against human papillomavirus types 16 and 18: follow-up from a randomised control trial. Lancet 2006;367(9518):1247–55.

60. Ang KK, Harris J, Wheeler R, et al. Human papillomavirus and survival of patients with oropharyngeal cancer. N Engl J Med 2010;363(1):24–35.

61. Lindel K, Beer KT, Laissue J, et al. Human papillomavirus positive squamous cell carcinoma of the oropharynx: a radiosensitive subgroup of head and neck carcinoma. Cancer 2001;92(4):805–13.
62. Fakhry C, Westra WH, Li S, et al. Improved survival of patients with human papillomavirus-positive head and neck squamous cell carcinoma in a prospective clinical trial. J Natl Cancer Inst 2008;100(4):261–9.
63. Cooper JS, Porter K, Mallin K, et al. National Cancer Database report on cancer of the head and neck: 10-year update. Head Neck 2009;31(6):748–58.
64. Hall SF, Groome PA, Irish J, et al. The natural history of patients with squamous cell carcinoma of the hypopharynx. Laryngoscope 2008;118(8):1362–71.
65. Zbaren P, Becker M, Lang H. Staging of laryngeal cancer: endoscopy, computed tomography and magnetic resonance versus histopathology. Eur Arch Otorhinolaryngol 1997;254(Suppl 1):S117–22.
66. Lefebvre JL, Chevalier D, Luboinski B, et al. Larynx preservation in pyriform sinus cancer: preliminary results of a European Organization for Research and Treatment of Cancer phase III trial. EORTC Head and Neck Cancer Cooperative Group. J Natl Cancer Inst 1996;88(13):890–9.
67. Terrell JE, Fisher SG, Wolf GT. Long-term quality of life after treatment of laryngeal cancer. The Veterans Affairs Laryngeal Cancer Study Group. Arch Otolaryngol Head Neck Surg 1998;124(9):964–71.
68. Boscolo-Rizzo P, Maronato F, Marchiori C, et al. Long-term quality of life after total laryngectomy and postoperative radiotherapy versus concurrent chemoradiotherapy for laryngeal preservation. Laryngoscope 2008;118(2):300–6.
69. Muscat JE, Wynder EL. Tobacco, alcohol, asbestos, and occupational risk factors for laryngeal cancer. Cancer 1992;69(9):2244–51.
70. Gissmann L, Wolnik L, Ikenberg H, et al. Human papillomavirus types 6 and 11 DNA sequences in genital and laryngeal papillomas and in some cervical cancers. Proc Natl Acad Sci U S A 1983;80(2):560–3.
71. Chu EA, Kim YJ. Laryngeal cancer: diagnosis and preoperative work-up. Otolaryngol Clin North Am 2008;41(4):673–95, v.
72. Cunnane M, Moore A, Harries M. Screening not staging: a retrospective study of the rate of synchronous primary malignancy in 44 T1/T2 laryngeal cancer in a tertiary head and neck unit. Clin Otolaryngol 2017;42(4):870–1.
73. Forastiere AA, Ismaila N, Wolf GT. Use of Larynx-Preservation Strategies in the Treatment of Laryngeal Cancer: American Society of Clinical Oncology Clinical Practice Guideline Update Summary. J Oncol Pract 2018;14(2):123–8.
74. Robertson D, Smith AJ. The microbiology of the acute dental abscess. J Med Microbiol 2009;58(Pt 2):155–62.
75. Safont M, Angelakis E, Richet H, et al. Bacterial lymphadenitis at a major referral hospital in France from 2008 to 2012. J Clin Microbiol 2014;52(4):1161–7.
76. Dorfman RF, Berry GJ. Kikuchi's histiocytic necrotizing lymphadenitis: an analysis of 108 cases with emphasis on differential diagnosis. Semin Diagn Pathol 1988; 5(4):329–45.
77. Dash GI, Kimmelman CP. Head and neck manifestations of sarcoidosis. Laryngoscope 1988;98(1):50–3.
78. Al-Khateeb TH, Al Zoubi F. Congenital neck masses: a descriptive retrospective study of 252 cases. J Oral Maxillofac Surg 2007;65(11):2242–7.
79. DeSanto LW. Laryngocele, laryngeal mucocele, large saccules, and laryngeal saccular cysts: a developmental spectrum. Laryngoscope 1974;84(8):1291–6.
80. Davison MJ, Morton RP, McIvor NP. Plunging ranula: clinical observations. Head Neck 1998;20(1):63–8.

# Update on Management of Hoarseness

Sandra Stinnett, MD[a],*, Monika Chmielewska, DO[b], Lee M. Akst, MD[c]

## KEYWORDS

- Hoarseness • Dysphonia • Laryngitis • Voice • Voice changes • Voice disturbances
- Laryngoscopy

## KEY POINTS

- Dysphonia generally describes any voice impairment; its cardinal symptom is hoarseness. Hoarseness is a symptom, not a diagnosis and is used to describe rough voice quality.
- History and physical examination are important in guiding the diagnosis of voice complaints; however, visualization of the larynx is essential for accurate diagnosis.
- Patients with dysphonia should be referred to an otolaryngologist if hoarseness persists beyond 4 weeks or if a serious underlying cause is suspected.
- The differential for dysphonia is broad and includes chronic laryngitis, glottic insufficiency, neoplasm, phonotraumatic lesions, and vocal fold motion impairment; a viral infection is most common.
- Empiric treatment in the absence of laryngeal examination is rarely indicated; evidence-based guidelines suggest instead that treatment be guided by laryngeal evaluation.

## SYMPTOMS

A detailed history regarding the patient's symptoms can offer many clues as to possible diagnosis and is the first step in evaluation of a patient with dysphonia.[1] There are several things to be considered when assessing symptoms of dysphonia, each discussed further herein. These include onset, nature of dysphonia, course of the dysphonia to date, associated complaints, and social history.

### Onset of Symptoms

Differentiating between acute and chronic onset of dysphonia can guide the clinician toward a possible etiology of the dysphonia. Sudden onset of dysphonia may reflect

Disclosure Statement: No disclosures.
[a] The University of Tennessee Health Science Center, Department of Otolaryngology-Head and Neck Surgery, 910 Madison Avenue, Suite 408, Memphis, TN 38163, USA; [b] ENT Associates, 3455 Regency Park Drive, Grand Blanc, MI 48439, USA; [c] Department of Otolaryngology–Head and Neck Surgery, Johns Hopkins University School of Medicine, 601 North Caroline Street, 6th Floor, Baltimore, MD 21287, USA
* Corresponding author.
E-mail address: sandrastinnettmd@gmail.com

Med Clin N Am 102 (2018) 1027–1040
https://doi.org/10.1016/j.mcna.2018.06.005
0025-7125/18/© 2018 Elsevier Inc. All rights reserved.

medical.theclinics.com

acute phonotraumatic lesion such as vocal fold hemorrhage or vocal fold polyp; many patients with vocal fold paralysis also experience sudden onset of voice complaints. In contrast, a gradual onset suggests possible slowly enlarging neoplasm, either benign or malignant, or chronic laryngeal inflammation.

Inquiring about the circumstances at time of onset of dysphonia also provide clues to the diagnosis. Did symptoms start after an upper respiratory tract infection? Did the patient have neck or thoracic surgery before the onset of symptoms? Were they intubated? All of these circumstances indicate a possible vocal fold paralysis, especially in a setting of a breathy voice. Has there been a new stressor in their life that correlates with onset of dysphonia? This finding indicates possible muscle tension dysphonia. Chronic sources of inflammation may include allergies, laryngopharyngeal reflux, or tobacco use. These patients may present with symptoms that have been present for several months to years with intermittent exacerbation.

### Nature of Dysphonia

Dysphonia may occur as the consequence of any disruption in vocal fold closure, vibration, or symmetry, although each of these physiologic problems may create a different voice issue. Listening critically and taking note of the quality of the voice during the history can help to guide the examiner to a differential diagnosis. Roughness most often indicates a lesion on the vibrating edge of the vocal fold, whereas a breathy or weak voice may reflect impaired vocal cord closure, as might occur with vocal fold paralysis. Pitch breaks and diplophonia (producing 2 frequencies at the same time) may indicate a large lesion on the vocal fold edge. A strained voice may indicate muscle tension dysphonia or spasmodic dysphonia. Assessing a patient's vocal quality is an aspect of the history that can begin the moment that the examiner starts their interaction with the patient.

### Course of Dysphonia

The progression of the dysphonia should be determined during the portion of the history. Are symptoms constant or intermittent? Does the patient return to a normal voice at any time? Has the dysphonia been stable since onset or gotten worse? Dysphonia that is intermittent or a patient who returns to a normal voice argues against a fixed lesion of the true vocal folds. Unremitting progression of the dysphonia over time should raise suspicion for a possible laryngeal malignancy that needs to be ruled out sooner than later.

### Other Associated Symptoms

The larynx plays important roles in breathing and swallowing in addition to its role in voice production. A complete history for any patient with dysphonia should include questions regarding dysphagia and dyspnea. If the patient coughs or chokes with liquids, it raises concern for glottis insufficiency such as might accompany vocal cord paralysis, and aspiration risk might prompt earlier referral. Mild solid food dysphagia, especially in the setting of globus pharyngeus, throat clearing, and dry cough may be associated with laryngopharyngeal reflux.[2] Persistent coughing during meals, significant weight loss, odynophagia, hematemesis, or a history of aspiration pneumonia should prompt more in-depth evaluation of swallowing function.

Some patients will be aware of their dysphonia enough to notice shortness of breath during phonation, with complaint that, "I run out of air when I speak." If this symptom is present, some form of glottic insufficiency such as a unilateral paralysis or paresis should be suspected in this situation. Other laryngeal pathologies, such as paradoxic vocal cord motion or laryngeal stenosis, may affect breathing as well, although the nature of the complaint is different; rather than "leaking air out," patients with obstruction to inhalation will complain of difficulty breathing in. The hallmark symptom of laryngeal involvement with restricted inhalation is stridor and any history of dyspnea with inhalational stridor should prompt referral for a laryngology evaluation.

Beyond breathing and swallowing function, other questions to ask a patient with dysphonia concern presence of neck mass, otalgia, or hemoptysis. If present, any of these might increase suspicion for malignancy.

### Social History

Taking a good social history allows for the examiner to gauge impact of dysphonia on the patient's overall quality of life. Also knowing a patient's voice use profile can help to estimate the risk for phonotraumatic lesions. Consider, for example, teachers who have a 20% to 50% lifetime incidence of dysphonia as compared with 6% to 15% for the general population.[3–6] Other high-risk professions include preachers, lawyers, and singers. Social history is also important insofar as tobacco and alcohol use are risk factors for malignancy.

## DIAGNOSTIC TESTING AND IMAGING STUDIES

Although the most important diagnostic test for a patient with dysphonia is laryngeal evaluation with laryngoscopy or videostroboscopy, there is a small role that laboratory testing and imaging studies might play for particular diagnoses. It is important to remember, though, that this testing is rarely indicated until these more specific diagnoses have been established.[7]

### Laryngoscopy

Laryngoscopy refers to visualization of the larynx. This examination can be done with a mirror, a flexible scope placed through the patient's nose, or a rigid telescope placed through the patient's mouth. These techniques are routinely available in most otolaryngology offices. In regular laryngoscopy, the vocal folds can be observed for lesions and motion of the vocal cords can be assessed as well. Diagnoses often made on laryngoscopy include exophytic lesions (polyps and/or tumors) and vocal cord paralysis. Contrary to some habituated practice patterns in which otolaryngologists diagnose reflux laryngitis on the basis of flexible laryngoscopy findings, there is no evidence to suggest that degree of redness or swelling of the larynx actually correlates with reflux as an etiology of dysphonia, although reflux might be suspected on the basis of history and confirmed through response to treatment or pH probe, the main benefit of laryngoscopy in this setting is in evaluation for nonreflux etiologies of dysphonia.[2,8–11]

### Stroboscopy

A videostroboscopic examination is a specialized type of laryngoscopy examination that uses a strobe light; in addition to viewing anatomy and motion, the use of a strobe light during the examination allows for a visual effect in which vocal cord vibration can be assessed as well. This examination, performed routinely by laryngologists (otolaryngologists who specialize in voice, swallowing, and airway disorders) and by some otolaryngologists as well, offers additional benefit of video-recording the examination for closer evaluation and playback. With an emphasis on function as well as structure and with brighter illumination and better optics, stroboscopy can sometimes identify etiologies for dysphonia that routine laryngoscopy might miss, for instance, small phonotraumatic lesions, subtle motion impairment (paresis), muscle tension dysphonia, and reduced vibration secondary to vocal cord scar or sulcus vocalis are all diagnoses that might be made on stroboscopy rather than on laryngoscopy. Although laryngoscopy is an important tool, videostroboscopy is considered the gold standard in the office evaluation of patients with dysphonia.

### Laboratory Testing

Laboratory testing is rarely obtained in the routine evaluation of dysphonia. Of course, some exceptions exist for particular diagnoses. For instance, if laryngoscopic examination leads to suspicion for an autoimmune condition causing dysphonia, then rheumatologic laboratory tests and inflammatory markers may be ordered. Generalized rheumatologic testing may include antineutrophil antibody titers, sedimentation rate, and C-reactive protein. More specific tests that may be ordered include antineutrophil cytoplasmic autoantibodies titers for granulomatosis with polyangiitis, which may present with subglottic stenosis. Rheumatoid factor is appropriate to evaluate for rheumatoid arthritis in the setting of cricoarytenoid joint fixation, and Sjogren's antibodies may be ordered to evaluate a sicca syndrome.

### Imaging

Imaging studies are not indicated in the setting of dysphonia before visualization of the larynx, because clinically they offer no benefit in the management of many common etiologies of dysphonia such as chronic laryngitis, phonotraumatic lesions, muscle tension dysphonia, and glottic insufficiency. If laryngoscopy reveals vocal cord paralysis that is otherwise unexplained (ie, onset does not coincide with neck surgery, for instance) or if a neoplasm is seen, then imaging is indicated. With suspected malignancy, a computed tomography scan of the neck can assess for the extent of the primary tumor and evaluate for cervical lymphadenopathy. For idiopathic vocal cord paralysis, the entire course of the recurrent laryngeal nerve should be imaged; this process may include computed tomography scans of both the neck and chest so that the inferior-most portions of the nerve can be seen as it wraps around the arch of the aorta (left) or subclavian artery (right) before reascending through the mediastinum into the neck to reach the larynx. A tumor anywhere along the course of the nerve can cause vocal cord paralysis, and imaging is done for this reason. Of note, evidence-based, multidisciplinary guidelines for the management of dysphonia explicitly suggest that ordering imaging for evaluation of dysphonia before diagnosis is not indicated.[7]

## DIFFERENTIAL DIAGNOSIS

There are many potential causes for dysphonia (**Table 1**); the rest of this section focuses on some of the most commonly encountered in clinical practice.

### Acute Laryngitis

Acute laryngitis is one of the most common causes of dysphonia. It is most commonly viral in origin, although acute laryngeal inflammation may also be secondary to vocal misuse or exposure to noxious agents. Viral inflammation of the vocal folds result in decreased vocal fold vibration, which produces a harsh, strained voice quality with decreased projection and increased effort. Stroboscopic findings consist of vocal fold edema and erythema, as well as reduced amplitude of the mucosal wave. Acute laryngitis is a self-limited process that usually lasts 2 weeks or less.

Treatment of acute laryngitis consists of implementing vocal hygiene techniques that include hydration, humidification and mucolytics. Routine antibiotic treatments are generally discouraged, unless there is evidence of bacterial superinfection.

**Table 1**
Differential diagnosis for hoarseness

| Phonotrauma and Benign Lesions | Neoplastic | Neurologic | Systemic Disease | Traumatic | Infectious | Structural Abnormalities | Other Causes |
|---|---|---|---|---|---|---|---|
| Nodules and other fibrous masses | Leukoplakia | Vocal fold paralysis and paresis | Granulomatosis with polyangiitis | External/internal trauma | Recurrent respiratory papillomatosis | Vascular malformations | Irritable larynx |
| Polyp | Squamous cell carcinoma | Spasmodic dysphonia | Relapsing polychondritis | Caustic injury | Bacterial laryngitis | Stenosis | Paradoxicl vocal fold motion |
| Varices/vascular lesions | Paraganglioma | Essential voice tremor | Syphilis | Scar/web | Fungal laryngitis | Laryngocele | Muscle tension dysphonia |
| Cyst | Granular cell tumor | Parkinson disease | Tuberculosis | | Viral laryngitis | Presbylarynges | Functional aphonia |
| Pseudocyst | | Postpolio syndrome | Rheumatoid laryngeal lesions | | Ulcerative laryngitis | | |
| Hemorrhage | | Myasthenia gravis | Amyloid | | | | |
| Granuloma | | | Sarcoid | | | | |
| Reinke edema | | | | | | | |
| Sulcus | | | | | | | |
| Scar | | | | | | | |

Bacterial and fungal infections, although rare, may be treated with antibiotics or antifungals when warranted. Amoxicillin-clavulanate (Augmentin) is the most commonly used antibiotic and fluconazole (Diflucan) is the antifungal that is often used. Corticosteroids are not commonly administered in the setting of acute laryngitis,[6] although exceptions are sometimes made for singers with performance obligations; in that setting, steroids may decrease inflammation and improve voice more quickly, although they do create a risk for vocal hemorrhage by aiding the performer in "pushing past" the inflammation. For this reason, vocal cord examination is recommended before empiric steroids are considered.

### Chronic Laryngitis

Chronic laryngitis involves a longer duration and is often caused by chemical irritation such as smoking, air pollutants, and inhalers, as well as mechanical irritations from traumatic cough or prolonged speaking. Other irritants include postnasal drip or laryngopharyngeal reflux. Because of its extensive etiopathology, chronic laryngitis is considered a nonspecific condition for prolonged laryngeal inflammation.[12]

Other than dysphonia, patients with chronic laryngitis may also report globus sensation, nonproductive cough, and a constant urge to clear the throat. Stroboscopic examination may reveal diffuse laryngeal edema and erythema and care must be taken to evaluate for concerning lesions such as leukoplakia. Treatment is contingent upon the cause of the inflammation. Primary measures include avoidance of noxious agents, such as cigarette smoke, as well as close surveillance of lesions suspicious for malignancy via stroboscopy. If patients report symptoms of reflux, such as heartburn, a trial of twice-daily proton pump inhibitors may be implemented for 2 months. Therapeutic lifestyle modifications such as reduction in caffeine consumption, carbonation, alcohol, and acidic foods should also be encouraged. Vocal hygiene is encouraged with reduced voice use and strategies to diminish throat clearing and coughing may help to reverse mechanical irritation. Other vocal hygiene tactics include increased hydration and humidification to decrease the viscosity of the glottic secretion.[13,14]

### Glottic Insufficiency

Glottic insufficiency is one of the most common contributing factor in patient who present with dysphonia. This usually results in breathy voice with limited projection and increased phonatory effort. The most common causes of glottic insufficiency resulting in dysphonia are:

1. Unilateral vocal fold paralysis,
2. Presbylaryngis (age-related atrophy of the vocal cords), and
3. Vocal fold paresis (unilateral vs bilateral).[15]

Unilateral vocal fold paralysis may be secondary to dysfunction of the brainstem nuclei, the vagus nerve, or the recurrent laryngeal nerve (**Fig. 1**). Evaluation includes identifying the cause. Iatrogenic nerve injury represents the most common cause for otolaryngologic referral. Common iatrogenic surgical causes include thyroidectomy/parathyroidectomy, anterior cervical disc surgery, esophagectomy, thymectomy, neck dissection, carotid endarterectomy, mediastinoscopy, and cardiothoracic surgery. Other nonsurgical iatrogenic causes include endotracheal intubation and less commonly prolonged nasogastric tube placement. Nonlaryngeal malignancies are another common cause, including cervical or thoracic neoplasms. In patients without a definitive surgical history explaining the paralysis, a computed tomography scan

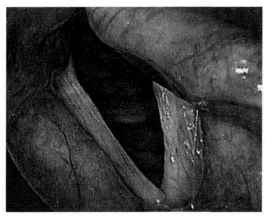

**Fig. 1.** Vocal fold paralysis of the left vocal fold, preventing from closing to midline and creating dysphonia.

should be obtained to address any lesions along the course of the recurrent laryngeal nerve from the skull base to mediastinum.[16]

If the patient's history suggests other possible causes (neurologic causes such as stroke or infectious causes such as Lyme disease) further blood work and imaging may be warranted. Other unusual causes include medications such as vinca alkaloids and systemic diseases such as sarcoidosis, rheumatoid arthritis, hypothyroidism, and gout.[17]

Patients with vocal fold paresis can have very subtle symptoms that may include loss of projection, vocal fatigue, loss of voice with increased use, odynophagia, loss of a portion of vocal range, and problems with singing voice. Videostroboscopy may reveal mild bowing of the vocal folds, incomplete glottic closure, or a prolonged open phase of the vibratory cycle. Laryngeal electromyography has not been proven to be diagnostic; however, some findings that are typically seen in paresis include reduced recruitment of motor units in the recurrent laryngeal nerve and superior laryngeal nerve distribution. Imaging studies are not considered useful in evaluating paresis, unless the paresis progressively worsens and/or becomes paretic. A neurologic consultation may be indicated to evaluate for conditions such as amyotrophic lateral sclerosis, postpolio syndrome, or pseudobulbar palsy.[18]

Presbylaryngis is known as the physiologic hoarseness of old age caused by senescent changes of the larynx. This process is not only attributed to vocal fold atrophy, but also to degeneration of the layers of the lamina propria as well. Presbylaryngis is found in 25% of individuals over 65 years old, affecting both men and women almost equally. The most common symptom is a thinned and strained voice with decreased projection and associated vocal fatigue with increased use. Laryngoscopic examination reveals bilateral vocal fold bowing and stroboscopy shows mild to moderate incomplete closure.[13]

### Benign Vocal Fold Lesions

Benign vocal fold lesions include nodules, polyp, cysts, fibrous masses, pseudocysts, and nonspecific lesions. Although the exact mechanism of the cause of benign vocal fold lesions is unknown, phonotrauma from vocal overuse and misuse is suspected to be the primary risk factor. This process results in shearing stresses during vocal fold vibration, particularly with vocal abuse resulting in cumulative phonotrauma.[18]

Vocal fold nodules are midmembranous fibrovascular callouses or scars that involve that superficial lamina propria as well as the basement membrane of the epithelium. They are usually symmetric, involve both vocal cords at the junction of the anterior one-third and posterior two-thirds of each cord. Stroboscopic findings demonstrate an hourglass-shaped closure with normal or minimally reduced mucosal wave.[18]

Polyps are usually unilateral exophytic or pedunculated lesions that extend from the vocal fold epithelium; however, a fibrous base may extend into the superficial lamina propria of the vocal fold on occasion. Stroboscopic finding again reveals an hourglass-shaped closure with little to no disturbance of the mucosal wave (**Fig. 2**). Intraoperative exploration may reveal a gelatinous material. Vocal fold cysts, in contrast, are subepithelial encapsulated lesions within the superficial aspect of the lamina propria. Cysts that are found near the vocal ligament and involve the deep aspect of the lamina propria. As a result, they have significant reduction of the mucosal wave on stroboscopy.

### Reinke's Edema

Reinke's edema, also known as polypoid corditis, is a benign condition of the vocal fold that involves accumulation of a gelatinous fluid throughout the superficial aspect of the lamina propria (**Fig. 3**). These accumulations can be severe, leading to airway obstruction, and may be asymmetric, although in general the disease process occurs throughout the entire vocal fold bilaterally, unlike the focal nature of a phonotraumatic polyp. It is commonly seen in patients with a long-term smoking history (97%); however, patients with severe laryngopharyngeal reflux and phonotrauma may also present with Reinke's edema.[13]

Patients typically present with progressive deepening of the voice in the fifth or sixth decade of life and a long history of smoking. Because these lesions are usually associated with significant smoking history, it is important to assess for any suspicious lesion that may need to be addressed; therefore, good visualization is necessary.[13]

### Recurrent Respiratory Papillomatosis

Recurrent respiratory papillomatosis is a benign neoplasm that is usually confined to the epithelium of the respiratory tract, most commonly the glottis (**Fig. 4**). Recurrent

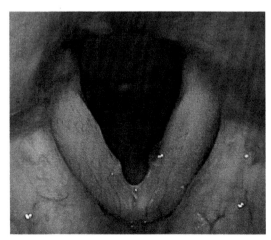

**Fig. 2.** A large right hemorrhagic polyp, resulting in impaired vocal fold vibration.

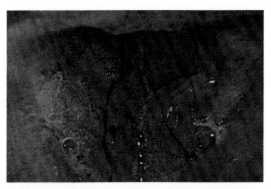

**Fig. 3.** Polypoid degeneration of the bilateral vocal folds, characteristic of Reinke's edema.

respiratory papillomatosis of the larynx is most commonly associated with human papilloma virus types 6 and 11. Human papilloma virus has a predisposition to histologic transitional zones, particularly where stratified squamous epithelium transitions to pseudostratified columnar epithelium, which explains why it is commonly found on the glottis. Patients usually present with a variety of symptoms that range from hoarseness to respiratory distress, contingent on the disease burden. On stroboscopy, the lesions are characteristically hypervascular, speckled fronds, although histologic confirmation is required for diagnosis.[19]

The goal of treatment is to decrease the disease burden by removing the papilloma and thus allowing for improved vocal function. However, even though the papillomas can be removed, the human papilloma virus itself remains in the tissue and recurrent growths are expected, as the name recurrent respiratory papillomatosis suggests. Repeated treatments might, therefore, be necessary, making it very important for long-term voice quality that there be efforts made to limit scar tissue and damage to normal vibration with each and every procedure.

### Leukoplakia

Leukoplakia of the vocal cords is usually characterized as a raised, white, plaquelike lesion on the epithelium of the vocal cords. Plaques may be singular in nature or diffuse along both vocal cords. Leukoplakia refers to the visual presentation of this

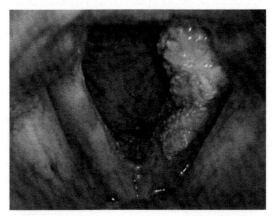

**Fig. 4.** Recurrent respiratory papillomatosis, whose presence along each vocal fold medial edge disrupts sound production.

disease process; histopathologically, the diagnosis of these plaques may range from benign keratosis to premalignant dysplasia, carcinoma in situ, or early malignancy. Leukoplakia may present with mild dysphonia or may be an incidental finding on head and neck examination. Early manifestations may take many years before progression to invasive carcinoma. Patients with leukoplakic lesions benefit from removal of the lesion, both to interfere with a natural history that may include progression to cancer and also to improve voice if the lesion is affecting vocal function. As with papilloma, leukoplakia is a superficial lesion and care should be taken operatively to limit damage to any associated normal tissue in the area of treatment. Serial evaluation with repeat treatment for recurrent disease may be necessary.[20]

### Vocal Cord Cancer

In 2014, an estimated 13,360 new cases of laryngeal cancer and 3660 deaths attributable to laryngeal cancer occurred in the United States. The annual incidence of laryngeal cancer is 3.1 cases per 100,000 for men and 1.0 cases per 100,000 for women. Smoking is the single greatest risk factor for laryngeal cancer, and excessive alcohol use has a synergistic effect as a risk factor. The most common symptoms associated with carcinoma of the vocal folds are hoarseness, change in pitch, and roughness of voice. The dysphonia associated with vocal fold carcinoma is constant and unremitting, unlike those caused by inflammatory disease processes. Odynophagia, dysphagia, otalgia, neck mass, unexplained weight loss, and hemoptysis increase the index of suspicion and are usually indicative of more advanced disease.[21]

Diagnosis is based on laryngeal examination and confirmed with biopsy. Videostroboscopic examination is helpful in predicting the depth of the lesion based on the degree of mucosal wave of the involved cord. Early glottic cancers can be treated successfully with either surgical excision or radiation therapy. T1 glottic cancer has a 5-year survival rate of 90% to 98%, with either of these treatment modalities. More advanced disease is usually treated with a combination of radiation therapy and surgery or chemotherapy.

### Neurologic Disorders and the Voice

Neurologic voice disorders are usually caused by abnormal control, coordination, or strength of the laryngeal muscles and vocal fold motion. Spasmodic dysphonia is a disorder of central motor processing that results in involuntary spasms that cause the excessive glottic closure (adductor spasmodic dysphonia) or inappropriate glottic opening (abductor spasmodic dysphonia) during speech. These processes result in either a strained–strangled speech pattern or breathy speech breaks, respectively. Interestingly, patients may not demonstrate speech breaks during singing or laughing tasks; however, symptoms may be exacerbated under physiologic stress. Spasmodic dysphonia typically presents in women in the fourth decade of life. Diagnosis is primarily based on auditory speech perception evaluation. Flexible laryngoscopic examination is supplementary and is done to rule out other lesions.[7]

Vocal tremor is distinct from laryngeal dystonia, because it involves tremor rather than spasm. Vocal tremor alone causes a tremulous voice quality without vocal breaks. Tremor may be visualized on phonation and with quiet respiration during laryngoscopic examination as well. Vocal tremor may exist alone or as part of an essential tremor. Essential tremor is a common movement disorder that usually involves the head, hands, and/or vocal tract.

Parkinson's disease is a neurodegenerative disease that can result in considerable disability. Classic clinical findings include bradykinesia, tremor, postural instability, and muscle rigidity. Phonatory symptoms include diminished projection and breathiness, as well as tremor. The voice is also monotone in quality. Associated dysphagia and dysarthria may also be present. Laryngoscopy may demonstrate vocal fold bowing. The voice component of Parkinson's disease is treated with voice therapy program called the Lee Silverman Voice Treatment with or without injection augmentation of the vocal folds to improve glottic configuration and closure.[7]

### Functional Voice Disorders

Functional voice disorders correlate with hyperfunctional dysphonia in the absence of specific anatomic disturbances, although anatomic and neurologic abnormalities may be present as well. The most common form of functional voice disorder is muscle tension dysphonia. Muscle tension dysphonia is associated with excessive and poorly regulated laryngeal muscle activity during speech. Muscle tension dysphonia can present as a primary hyperfunction often associated with onset after an upper respiratory tract infection, inappropriate pitch use, reflux, or significant voice demand. It may also present as a secondary compensatory mechanism for glottic insufficiency. Patients may also complain of odynophonia, mostly with prolonged speaking, owing to significant tension of the supraglottic muscles.[12]

## TREATMENT AND MANAGEMENT

Treatment for dysphonia is contingent upon the underlying diagnosis. With that in mind and understanding the importance of laryngoscopy and/or videostroboscopy in creating the appropriate differential diagnosis by visualizing the vocal folds, the most important thing that a nonotolaryngologist may need to know about dysphonia is when to refer a patient for laryngeal evaluation. Laryngoscopy is indicated for the assessment of hoarseness if symptoms do not improve or resolve within 4 weeks or if there is a suspected underlying serious condition. Hoarseness persisting after 4 weeks is unlikely to resolve on its own and requires special attention to appropriately diagnose and treat. Serious conditions are those characterized by a potential decrease in lifespan or significantly impacting their quality of life, such as malignancy.[22,23] Symptoms that should increase a clinician's index of suspicion for serious lesion include a history of tobacco or alcohol use, neck mass, otalgia, hemoptysis, difficulty breathing or stridor, and unexplained weight loss. Patients who experience hoarseness after recent intubation or head and neck surgery should also undergo videostroboscopy.

Once the diagnosis has been made, treatment may be indicated. Specific approaches to treatment of each etiology of dysphonia are discussed in the Differential Diagnosis, elsewhere in this article; this section discusses general treatment approaches more broadly. The treatment modalities to be considered are behavioral, pharmacologic, and surgical.

### Behavioral Interventions

Behavioral Interventions include vocal hygiene and voice therapy. As discussed, vocal hygiene includes increased hydration and humidification to reduce the viscosity of glottic secretions. This measure will provide significant glottic lubrication and help to alleviate hoarseness, barring any other lesions being present. Often, voice rest may be indicated and has been found to be useful in short periods of time to help resolve edema and inflammatory changes that may be secondary to mechanical irritation or trauma.[12]

Voice therapy is useful to assist with teaching and implementing various techniques that are aimed at minimizing the mechanical insults and harmful behaviors. The speech–language pathologist plays an important role in the diagnostic and therapeutic team needed for quality voice care. Voice therapy is considered essential for effective management of benign vocal fold lesions and functional voice disorders.[12]

### Pharmacologic Interventions

Pharmacologic interventions may be beneficial in managing certain causes of hoarseness. The role of antireflux medications remains to be elucidated in the management of dysphonia. The main issue is the heterogeneity in diagnostic criteria for laryngopharyngeal reflux, which poses a great hindrance in future prospective outcomes studies. Often, patients who present with chronic laryngitis reports symptoms of heartburn and may benefit from a 2-month trial of twice daily proton pump inhibition.[22,23] In patients with vocal process granulomas, proton pump inhibitors have been used to reduce irritation to the area of exposed cartilage, and repetitive phonotrauma. This measure, in conjunction with inhaled corticosteroids, has been found to be helpful in the management of vocal process granulomas.[6]

Patients who suffer from vocal tremor associated with essential tremor may respond to the medications that treat the essential tremor. These agents include anxiolytics and beta-blockers, which would not result in worsening hypophonia associated with other interventions, such as botulinum toxin (Botox) injections. It is important to note that there is no clear defined role for systemic steroids in treating hoarseness currently.[24]

Botulinum toxin is used in the setting of spasmodic dysphonia and is usually performed in office in conjunction with electromyography. Injecting botulinum toxin into appropriate laryngeal muscles can weaken these muscles and reduce the associated spasm. It may also result in reduced amplitude of the tremor; however, it may exacerbate hypophonia in these patients.[24]

### Surgical Interventions

Surgery for hoarseness is always aimed at restoring or preserving the normal physiology of phonation. Microlaryngoscopy is one of the mainstay surgical procedure in modern laryngology and is used in conjunction with various other surgical techniques, such as laser excision or the cold technique, for the removal of vocal fold lesions and for pathologic diagnosis. Vocal fold augmentation is indicated for patients with dysphonia secondary to vocal fold paralysis or significant presbylaryngis. Augmentation, known as injection laryngoplasty, uses a variety of temporary fillers that medialize the immobile or atrophied cord, lasting from 4 weeks to 18 months. Patients with permanent vocal fold paralysis or severe presbylaryngis may undergo a more permanent augmentation procedure, known as medialization thyroplasty, with Gortex or sialistic implant.[25]

As technological advancements are made and innovativeness continues to excel, in-office procedures are becoming more and more common. Injection laryngoplasty, laser excision of leukoplakia and/or recurrent respiratory papillomatosis, and biopsy may be performed as in-office procedures. There are many benefits to an in-office procedure if the patient is able to tolerate it that include the lack of general anesthesia, shorter duration of the procedure, and no requirement for any activity restriction after the procedure is completed.[25]

Benign vocal fold lesions that do not respond to voice therapy may undergo phonosurgery with the primary goal being to remove the lesion that impairs vibration while preserving the remaining, pliable speech language pathologist (SLP) and restore vocal fold vibration.

The advent of microlaryngeal surgery has revolutionized the management of many laryngeal disease entities that cause hoarseness with particular emphasis on voice preservation. There are several key principals in maximizing positive outcomes in microlaryngeal surgery. Optimal intraoperative visualization is key to properly assess vocal fold lesions and to create a surgical plan that will allow for maximum voice preservation. Specialists in laryngeal surgery often have special laryngoscopes and operative tools that help them to prioritize preservation of laryngeal function in phonosurgery. Care must be taken to excise the lesion while preserving laryngeal function and therefore likely improving phonation in patients with benign vocal fold lesions. In patients with suspected or known malignancy, there is a fine balance between voice preservation versus oncologic resection with adequate margins, the latter being the primary goal while keeping the prior in mind.[26] This theory holds true for excision of recurrent respiratory papillomatosis lesions as well. It is important to note that patients with recurrent respiratory papillomatosis or cancer/leukoplakia require close surveillance by an otolaryngologist for serial monitoring.[25]

## SUMMARY

Hoarseness is a common presenting complaint that may be a symptom of a large spectrum of diseases, both benign and malignant. An understanding of the anatomy and physiology of normal voice production as well as a thorough history and examination is essential. Diagnoses are as simple as acute laryngitis, which is self-limited, or as complex as recurrent respiratory papillomatosis and malignancy, requiring repeat excisions and close surveillance. The aim of all treatment is to optimize phonatory function and often to restore a patent airway. If there are any concerns, referral to otolaryngology for laryngoscopy is of the utmost importance for prompt diagnoses and treatment initiation.

## REFERENCES

1. Titze IR, Lemke J, Montequin D. Populations in the U.S. workforce who rely on voice as primary tool of trade: a preliminary report. J Voice 1997;11:254-9.
2. Gooi Z, Ishman SL, Bock JM, et al. Laryngopharyngeal reflux: paradigms for evaluation, diagnosis and treatment. Ann Otol Rhinol Laryngol 2014;123(10):677-85.
3. Smith E, Gray M, Dove S. Frequency and effects of teachers voice problems. J Voice 1997;11:81-7.
4. Mattiske JA, Oates MJ, Greenwood KM. Vocal problems among teachers: a review of prevalence, causes, prevention, and treatments. J Voice 1998;12:489-99.
5. Simberg S, Laine A, Sala E, et al. Prevalence of voice disorders among future teachers. J Voice 2000;14:231-5.
6. Roy N, Merill RM, Thibeault S, et al. Prevalence of voice disorders in teachers and general population. J Voice 2004;47:281-93.
7. Stachler R, Francis D, Schwatrz S, et al. Clinical practice guideline: hoarseness (dysphonia) (update). Otolaryngol Head Neck Surg 2018;158(1):S1-42.
8. Akst LM, Hague OJ, Clarke JO, et al. The changing impact of gastroesophageal reflux disease in clinical practice. Ann Otol Rhinol Laryngol 2017;126(3):229-35.
9. Dhillon VK, Akst LM. How to approach laryngopharyngeal reflux: an otolaryngology perspective. Curr Gastroenterol Rep 2016;18(8):44.
10. Fritz MA, Persky MJ, Fang Y, et al. The accuracy of the laryngopharyngeal reflux diagnosis: utility of the stroboscopic exam. Otolaryngol Head Neck Surg 2016; 155(4):629-34.

11. Gooi Z, Ishman SL, Bock JM, et al. Changing patterns in reflux care: 10-year comparison of ABEA members. Ann Otol Rhinol Laryngol 2015;124(12):940–6.
12. Reiter R, Hoffman TK, Pichard A, et al. Hoarseness – causes and treatments. Dtsch Arztebl Int 2015;112:329–37.
13. Zeitels SM, Casiano RR, Gardner GM, et al. Management of common voice problems: committee report. Otolaryngol Head Neck Surg 2002;126:333–48.
14. Akst L. Hoarseness and laryngitis. In: Bope ET, Rakel RE, Kellerman RD, editors. Conn's current therapy. 17th edition. Philadelphia: Saunders Elsevier; 2010. p. 225–6.
15. Swibel Rosenthal LH, Benninger MS, Deeb RH. Vocal fold immobility: a longitudinal analysis of etiology over 20 years. Laryngoscope 2007;117:1864–70.
16. Benninger MS, Gillen JB, Altman JS. Changing etiology of vocal fold immobility. Laryngoscope 1998;108:1346–9.
17. Pardo-Maza A, Garcia-Lopez I, Santiago-Perez S, et al. Laryngeal electromyography for prognosis of vocal fold paralysis. J Voice 2017;31:90–3.
18. Naunheim MR, Carroll TL. Benign vocal fold lesions: update on nomenclature, cause, diagnosis and treatment. Curr Opin Otolaryngol Head Neck Surg 2017; 25:453–8.
19. Cicenia J, Almeida FA. Recurrent respiratory papillomatosis. In: Mehta A, Jain P, Gildea T, editors. Diseases of the central airways. Respiratory medicine. Cham (Switzerland): Humana Press; 2016. p. 215–29.
20. Parker NP. Vocal fold leukoplakia: incidence, management and prevention. Curr Opin Otolaryngol Head Neck Surg 2017;25:464–8.
21. Gale N, Zidar N, Cardesa A, et al. Benign and potentially malignant lesions of the squamous epithelium and squamous cell carcinoma. In: Cardesa A, Slootweg P, Gale N, et al, editors. Pathology of the head and neck. Berlin: Springer; 2016. p. 1–48.
22. Schwartz SR, Cohen SM, Dailey SH, et al. Clinical practice guideline: hoarseness (Dysphonia). Otolaryngol Head Neck Surg 2009;141:S1–31.
23. Karatayli-Ozgursoy S, Pacheco-Lopez P, Hillel AT, et al. Laryngeal dysplasia, demographics and treatment: single-institution, 20 year review. JAMA Otolaryngol Head Neck Surg 2015;141:313–8.
24. Thekdi AA, Rosen CA. Surgical treatment of benign vocal fold lesions. Curr Opin Otolaryngol Head Neck Surg 2003;10:492–6.
25. Zeitels SM, Healy GB. Laryngology and phonosurgery. N Engl J Med 2003;349: 882–92.
26. Merati AL, Heman-Ackah YD, Abaza M, et al. Common movement disorders affecting the larynx: a report from the neurolaryngology committee of the AAO-HNS. Otolaryngol Head Neck Surg 2005;133:654–65.

# The Aging Face

Anil R. Shah, MD*, Paige M. Kennedy, MD

## KEYWORDS

- Facial aging • Antiaging • Rhytids • Laser therapy • Implants • Fillers
- Cosmetic surgery

## KEY POINTS

- The aging face is a popular topic in modern medicine, and the process of aging is discussed in this article.
- To understand and treat unwanted signs of aging, it is imperative to understand the biological and physical causes of facial aging, the contributing factors to facial aging, preventative measures to avoid advanced facial aging, and the current treatment options.
- Changes to the human face are progressive with time; however, there are many methods, both surgical and nonsurgical, to reduce the stigmata of aging and provide patients with the appearance they desire.

## CAUSE AND EFFECTS OF FACIAL AGING

The causes and effects of the aging face have been studied extensively over the last decade. A better understanding of how we age and the resultant changes have allowed patients to reap the rewards with a full gamut of treatment options. For physicians to properly treat the aging face, one must first understand the processes of senescence. The advances in both surgery and medicine have helped to create a more comprehensive approach to the aging face.

Skin has classically 2 different types of changes seen in aging, divided into intrinsic aging and extrinsic aging. Intrinsic aging occurs as a result of the normal aging phenomenon. Extrinsic aging is typically due to photoaging, commonly secondary to excessive sun exposure; however, other processes such as gravity and smoking play a role in the aging of the face.

If we think of young skin as a lush thick forest, the converse would be withered, dry desert. As our skin ages, our skin as a whole thins. Thinning of the epidermis is thought to occur in part owing to the flattening of the rete ridge pattern.[1] The dermis of the skin

The authors have no commercial or financial conflicts of interest and no funding sources to disclose.
Department of Otolaryngology–Head and Neck Surgery, The University of Chicago Medicine, The University of Chicago Medicine and Biological Sciences, 5841 South Maryland Avenue, Room E-103, MC1035, Chicago, IL 60637, USA
* Corresponding author. 845 North Michigan Avenue, Suite 934E, Chicago, IL 60611.
E-mail address: shah@shahfacialplastics.com

also thins, in addition to the subcutaneous tissue. The dermis and epidermal junction become flattened, a source of impaired nutrient transfer.

The overall thinning of the skin results in slower wound healing and increased skin fragility. Epidermal cell turnover is impaired, resulting in less effective desquamation of the skin. When we are younger, our skin cells turnover roughly every 20 days. As we age, the shedding of our skin slows down, taking as long as 30 or more days for new skin cells to replenish.[2]

The overall composition of the skin is changed as well with a higher ratio of type III collagen to type I collagen. Much of the collagen present becomes fragmented. Overall collagen is also reduced in part owing to reduced fibroblasts. Some studies demonstrate that the overall collagen content per unit area of skin surface decreases by approximately 1% per year, leaving the skin with both a loss of collagen and an alteration in the ratio of skin components.[3]

Extrinsic causes of aging skin are most often attributed to photoaging. Whereas intrinsic aging is a thinning of skin and slowing down of its cells, extrinsic aging is damaged skin seen all the way down to subcellular messenger RNA. Elastosis occurs, which is the accumulation of elastin material below the epidermal–dermal junction. In photoaging, the epidermis does thin, but there is more chaos in the structure. Photoaged skin often has more fragmentation of collagen and elastin.[4]

Langerhans cells are cells within the epidermal basal layer and spinous layer that function in the pathogenesis of dermatoses as well as in neoplastic processes. Langerhans cells play a role in immune surveillance of the skin. It has been observed that, with time, skim immunity decreases, as is seen in elderly skin that becomes more susceptible to skin cancers, as well as an increased susceptibility to infections of the skin. As time goes on, the quality of Langerhans cells within ultraviolet light–exposed skin has been noted to decrease, as the cells become smaller and have shorter and poorly branched dendrites. These changes are thought to make the cells less functional as immune cells, thereby increasing skin susceptibility to neoplastic processes.[5]

## FACIAL CHANGES WITH AGING

The fundamental shape of our face changes with age as a result of alteration of the soft tissues, skeletal support, and changes of the skin. The skin becomes wrinkled, less elastic, and more irregular, and the surface becomes more discolored. Soft tissues of the face descend with gravity and muscular atrophy over time. Bone loss occurs in the facial skeleton, and is as much evident in the face as it is in other areas of the body.

The aging process results in the brow and forehead area elongating in the upper one-third of the hairline as the brow recedes and hairline recession takes place. Brow ptosis is common and can create hooding of the lateral brow, which gives the appearance of darkening of the area surrounding the eye. This phenomenon is a result of increased skin laxity after a loss of elastin in the skin matrix, as well as gravitational changes. The constant contraction of the orbicularis oculi muscle can contribute as well.

The periorbital area results in several changes. First of all, excessive skin from the lid can be seen as a combination of brow descent and a loss of skin elasticity. Patient's experience 2 phenomena: dermatochalasis, a term for excessive skin in the upper and lower eyelid (baggy eyes), and blepharochalasis, which is inflammation of the eyelids leading to fluctuating degrees of edema, stretching the skin and causing redundant tissue to form over the eyelids. Ptosis can be seen in some patients and results from the levator muscle, the levator aponeurosis, to slightly separate with age. Many of these changes occur in concert with predictable skeletal changes. These changes can help us to identify in a skull the difference between a 20-year-old and an 80-year-old. The orbital width increases with age. An overall contour change occurs as well, with an increase in height in the superior orbital rim medially as well as in the inferior orbital rim laterally. This better understanding has led to less removal of fat in blepharoplasty than in previous years. Loss of fat in this region can also lead to wasting of the temples, leading to a gaunt appearance.[6,7]

Aging of the midface results in overall drooping of the soft tissues, in particular the orbicularis oculi and malar soft tissue complex. The descent of these tissues in part leads to a deepening of the smile lines or the nasolabial folds. The volumetric loss here can result in an overall hollowing of the face from a combination of loss of fat as well as loss of maxillary and alveolar height (**Fig. 1**).[8]

The nose typically becomes longer and seems to be more drooped with time. The skin of the nose thins with aging, and can occasionally reveal bony or cartilaginous abnormalities not noticed previously. The nose loses support, or tip projection, leading to a drooped appearance. The weakening of nasal ligaments also contributes and the ptotic tip can lead to issues with function and appearance. The loss of maxillary and alveolar bone can lead to further loss of tip support.[9]

The lower face results in an excess of tissues seen as a result of a combination of factors. This result can lead to a fullness of tissue along the jaw, called jowls. The loss of mandibular bone can lead to changes as well, including a decrease in chin projection and enhancement of the prejowl sulcus. The chin can alter over time as well. Typically, a combination of loss of bone along the mandible, coupled with loss of soft tissue of the chin, can create descent of the chin and loss of projection. A witch's

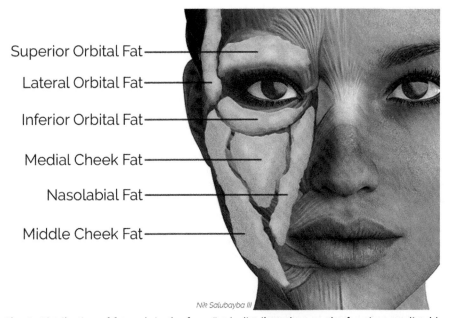

Superior Orbital Fat

Lateral Orbital Fat

Inferior Orbital Fat

Medial Cheek Fat

Nasolabial Fat

Middle Cheek Fat

Nik Salubayba III

**Fig. 1.** Distribution of fat pads in the face. Fat is distributed across the face in a predictable pattern. Over time, these areas begin to atrophy and descend. Augmentation of these fat pads, as well as suspension techniques, can give the face a more youthful appearance.

chin deformity occurs when the crease is overly prominent owing to descent of the soft tissues of the chin coupled with excessive fullness of the submentum.[10,11]

The perioral area results in an overall longer upper lip with finer lines, such as smoker lines, present. The overall longer lip elongation results from a combination of thinning of the red lip with elastic changes resulting in enhancement of the white lip. The fine rhytides are a combination of the orbicularis oris muscle weakening, as well as thinning of the skin surrounding the lips.

The neck results in a variety of changes owing to a combination of a loss of skin elasticity and a loss of volume of the neck, as well as gravitational changes of the muscle and skin. The supporting structures of the neck, including the mandible and chin, often weaken over time, contributing to the lax appearance of the neck. The loss of volume and gradual thinning of the skin of the neck can lead to the visibility of platysmal bands.[10] Platysmal bands are thought to also occur from separation along the midline, creating 2 bands of muscle to the neck rather than a unified muscular attachment.[12]

Earlobes can change as well, with elongation noted along the ears. Weakening of the ligaments of the ear and a loss of volume in the earlobe can cause earlobes to look flaccid and stretched. Longer earlobes are particularly an issue with women wearing heavier earrings.

## SOLUTIONS TO THE AGING FACE
### Topicals and Diet

Before using cosmeceuticals or surgical interventions as antiaging strategies, there are preventative measures that can be taken to promote youthful skin. Two important ways to slow facial aging are topical interventions, such as exfoliation and cleansing of the face, as well as the use of sunscreen. A second nonprocedural method of promoting skin health is maintaining a balanced diet. With regard to using sunscreen, it is well-described that ultraviolet irradiation contributes significantly to cutaneous photoaging. Preventing ultraviolet A and ultraviolet B irradiation reacting with the skin components, such as keratinocytes, is a preventative method to avoid skin damage and sustain a youthful appearance.[13] Other topical solutions to preventing facial aging include retinoids. Retinoids encompasses retinol, or vitamin A, and its natural and synthetic derivatives. Natural retinoids include retinol, retinyl esters, retinal, and retinoic acid. In cosmetic therapy, the most frequently used retinoids are retinyl palmitate and retinyl acetate. These esters are stored in keratinocytes once applied to the skin and they work to abolish cellular atypia and increase the compaction of the layer of skin known as the stratum corneum. These molecules also function to inhibit the effects of metalloproteinases, which are known to cause the degradation of collagen and elastin, typically for the function of wound healing; however, this activity leads to inflammation and photoaging as well.[14,15]

With regard to diet, the data suggest that caloric restriction and fasting cycles may decrease the production of hormones involved in expediting the aging process. Antioxidants and vitamins are associated with contributing to the repair of photodamage to improve the appearance of photoaged skin.[16]

### Medical Interventions

#### Hormone therapy

One important strategy to antiaging is hormone therapy. As both males and females age, their levels of hormones secreted from the pituitary gland, adrenals, and gonads decrease. These decreases contribute to skin aging, as well as decreased lean body mass, sexual desire, intellectual function, and mood. Hormone replacement therapy has been shown to aid in reducing the decline of the previously mentioned domains.[17,18] In regards to skin aging, dehydroepiandrosterone and its sulfate ester dehydroepiandrosterone sulfate have been used to improve hydration, skin thickness, sebum production, and pigmentation.[19] Another hormone used to improve skin appearance with aging is estrogen. Estrogen levels peak in the mid to late 20s in women and begins to decrease by approximately 50% in the 50s. These levels continue to decrease through menopause. Estrogen is a hormone that is associated with maintaining a youthful appearance by improving skin tone and pigmentation, and decreasing the appearance of wrinkles. Estrogen oral therapy given as oral conjugated equine estrogens is used to improve skin health.[20] The use of extrinsic hormonal therapy must be driven by experts and should be limited to use in a medical setting, because exogenous hormone use has been suggested to cause unwanted cell proliferation.

### Platelet-rich plasma

Platelet-rich plasma (PRP) is a derivative of whole blood in which the patient's blood is centrifuged to remove red blood cells, leaving a concentrate of PRP protein. This solution contains a condensed concentration of growth factors. PRP works by releasing platelet alpha granules, which in turn promote an upsurge in growth factors and cytokines to the area of interest. PRP is used across a wide range of specialties. In facial plastic surgery, PRP is used as an adjunctive therapy, playing a role in many areas of regenerative medicine including orthopedics, hair restoration, and aesthetic medicine. More recently, PRP has been used with fat transfer for enrichment, as well as with fillers to help enhance their overall impact. A recent study found that PRP-assisted fat resulted in superior volume maintenance over time compared with a control group. The mechanism of action is believed to be in part owing to the enhancement of angiogenesis and cell proliferation associated with PRP.[21] The use of PRP in combination with hyaluronic acid has been reported in patients with knee osteoarthritis to be superior to hyaluronic acid alone.[22] The use in facial aesthetics and aging has been used by the senior author and anecdotally has noted increased duration and integration into tissues.

### Lasers

LASER therapy is used on facial skin for skin resurfacing. Specific wavelengths are used to create a controlled injury to the face. In varying degrees, all lasers work to improve the appearance of fine lines and photoaging, as well as to soften scarring and smooth dyspigmentation. There are 5 major lasers used on the skin: ablative and nonablative lasers that have both fractionated and unfractionated forms, and radiofrequency lasers. Ablative lasers vaporize tissue, removing the epidermal layer, and are considered more aggressive than nonablative lasers. Damage to the epidermal layer promotes collagen formation and dermal retraction, which gives the skin a more tightened appearance. Nonablative lasers leave the epidermis intact. Nonfractionated lasers act on the entire surface area of the skin. Fractionated lasers target a portion of the projected area of the skin undergoing treatment.

Laser use began with the $CO_2$ laser, an ablative laser. This laser works at the 10,600-nm wavelength to selectively ablate the skin. The erbium laser is also an ablative laser and works at the wavelength of 2940 nm. The $CO_2$ laser effects skin at a depth of 100 to 150 μm layer of tissue, whereas the erbium YAG laser has an absorption coefficient 16 times greater than the $CO_2$ laser, causing a decrease in the penetration depth by a factor of 10 when compared with the $CO_2$ laser. Using the wound healing model in laser recuperation, the skin goes through the stages of erythema, proliferation, and remodeling over a period of 1 year.[23] Patients must be instructed that results after laser resurfacing are often cumulative and that the final results take time.

Picosecond (PICO) lasers are a different type of laser that use a faster pulse (trillionth of a second) versus conventional lasers (billionth of a second). The speed of the PICO laser allows for patients with difficult-to-treat conditions, such as hyperpigmentation and melasma, to be treated more effectively than with other types of lasers by imparting less heat to the area. The PICO laser can also be used with a fractional lens to create laser-induced optical breakdown, which are a controlled injury response to the laser itself.[24] Choosing the type of laser therapy in each situation requires taking the patient, risk factors, and desired results into careful consideration.

### Facial fillers

Facial fillers are a variety of biologic and synthetic materials that are injected into the face to correct lines and wrinkles and to augment the face. Fillers ideally should be biocompatible, hypoallergenic, nontoxic, noncarcinogenic, and provide a long-lasting result over time.

Currently, there are several categories of fillers approved by the US Food and Drug Administration (**Table 1**). The largest category of fillers are hyaluronic acid fillers. The hyaluronic acid products vary by the amount of cross-linking and particle size. By varying these variables, products can have either a high G' (stiffer product) or thinner G' product. Higher G' products are best for deeper applications, such as the nasolabial fold and facial augmentation. Lower G' products are best for superficial lines, lips, and tear troughs.[25] The main advantage of hyaluronic acid products is reversibility with the enzyme hyaluronidase.

Other categories of fillers include calcium hydroxyapatite, poly-L-lactic acid (PLLA), and polymethyl methacrylate. Calcium hydroxyapatite (Radiesse) is a thicker product that is approved for nasal labial folds and lasts up to 18 months. PLLA (Sculptra) lasts for up to 2 years and is thought to work by the PLLA particles stimulating fibroblasts to produce collagen, creating volume as the PLLA is degraded and respired as $CO_2$.[26] Polymethyl methacrylate (Bellafil) is approved by the US Food and Drug Administration for nasal labial folds and works by injection of synthetic polymethyl methacrylate microspheres into the body, allowing it to last for 5 years and even longer.

There are several complications seen with fillers. Edema, ecchymosis, and asymmetry can be mitigated by technique. Granuloma and nodule formation can occur as a result of multinucleated giant cells and can occur with any facial filler.[27] Embolism of fillers has been reported and can cause soft tissue necrosis, central retinal arterial occlusion, and cerebral ischemia.[28] The use of cannulas and low-pressure injections, as well as avoiding boluses have been proposed mechanisms to decrease the probability of occurrence.

The molecular basis of these fillers are different; however, each aims to aid in facial augmentation and filling areas of deep lines or tissue loss, with varying durations of effect.

### Neuromodulators

Neuromodulators are made of the exotoxin botulinum, which is produced by the bacteria *Clostridium botulinum* (**Table 2**). There are 9 toxins that are known, but only toxins A and B are commercially available for use. Botulinum toxin (Botox) works by binding to the presynaptic vesicles and preventing the release of acetylcholine. The effect takes approximately 1 week to see a temporary paralysis lasting up to 4 months as

**Table 1**
**Formulations of commercially available facial fillers**

| Filler | Brand Name | Use | Duration of Effect |
|---|---|---|---|
| NASHA (nonanimal Streptococci hyaluronic acid) | Restylane/ Juvederm/ Belotero | Fine lines/moderate wrinkles and facial augmentation | 6–24 mo |
| Calcium hydroxlyapatite | Radiesse | Moderate to deep skin folds | 6–12 mo |
| Poly-L-lactic acid | Sculptra | Severe folds and facial augmentation | 2 y |
| Polymethyl methacrylate | Bellafil | Moderate to severe nasolabial folds | 5 years–permanent |

the body regenerates new SNAP-25 nerve terminals.[29] The main complications with botulinum toxin are brow ptosis, lid ptosis, bruising, and facial asymmetry.

Neuromodulators vary in exact composition, however they all work in relaxing muscles of the face to improve the appearance of lines of facial aging, with variances in dosage and effect.

## Surgical Interventions

### Brow lift
The brow can be elevated with a variety of techniques, including coronal and endoscopic brow lifts, as well as lateral brow lift via temporal incision. The coronal brow lift has lost favor over time because it involves a large scar in a coronal pattern within the scalp. The coronal brow lift can lengthen the upper one-third of the face and lead to a loss of sensation. The endoscopic brow lift can be used to camouflage incisions in the hairline and provide less drastic recovery than the traditional coronal approach. The lateral brow lift is a minimally invasive approach hiding an incision in the temporal areas of the scalp and can lift the lateral brow only.[30]

### Eye lift
Blepharoplasty can occur on either the upper or lower eyelid and is designed to remove either fat or excessive skin from the area. Upper lid blepharoplasty is performed by hiding an incision in the supratarsal crease and removing excessive skin and/or fat from the lid to prevent excessive hooding of the lid. Overzealous removal of skin can lead to dry eyes, lagophthalmus, and other complications.

Lower lid blepharoplasty is performed by removing either fat or skin or both from the lower eyelid area. Periorbital fat from the lower eye area can be removed via an internal approach (transconjunctival) or external approach (subciliary). The main advantage of the transconjunctival approach is avoidance of an external scar as well as avoidance

**Table 2**
**Neuromodulators by the US Food and Drug Administration**

| Neuromodulator | Brand Name | Use |
|---|---|---|
| Onabotulinumtoxin A | Botox | Glabellar and lateral canthal lines |
| AbobtulinumtoxinA | Dysport | Glabellar lines |
| Incobotulinumtoxin A | Xeomin | Glabellar lines |
| Rimabotulinumtoxin B | Myobloc | Not often used, no indication |

of lower lid malposition. The subciliary approach is used when excessive skin is seen in the lower lid. Skin is excised from the lower lid, paying special attention to avoid excessive removal of skin, which can lead to ectropion.[31]

### Nasal lift

Rhinoplasty on the aging individual bears special attention. Individuals with well-established identities should avoid drastic changes to allow for a better preservation of self. The nose is often supported to reduce overall nasal length with further refinements in nasal tip and improved airflow as desired outcomes as well.[32]

### Chin augmentation

Chin augmentation must balance the existing facial, features including the nose and forehead. Most often, a line drawn perpendicular to the lower lip represents the ideal position of the chin for men, and a line drawn 1 to 2 mm behind this is ideal for women. However, for patients with an aging face, chin augmentation should take place in the context of matching the chin proportions to the appearance of the chin they had in their 20s. Chin implants can be placed either through a submental or intraoral incision and offer a permanent solution to chin support. The main risks of chin augmentation are infection and extrusion, which can be minimized with sterile techniques. Permanent sensory nerve damage can similarly be avoided by surgeon's knowledge of the underlying anatomy.[33]

### Midface lift

The midface lift can be performed in isolation with an endoscopic approach or in combination with a facelift. The midface lift focuses on suspending the malar fat pad in a superior lateral direction. Often, the skin of the lower eyelid bunches along the lower lateral eyelid with the surgeon removing excessive skin. Over time, descension of the midface can cause the lower eyelid to descend, resulting in ectropion. The midface lift has an additional risk of potential injury to the buccal and zygomatic branches of the facial nerve.[34]

### Rhytidectomy

Rhytidectomy involves the improvement of face and/or neck to help visibly lift either the muscle or the skin of the face. An incision is typically started in the temporal hairline and extended to either in front of the ear (pretragal) or behind the ear (posttragal) position before extending into the posterior hairline. There are a variety of approaches to lift the face including superficial muscular aponeurotic system (SMAS) lifts, subperiosteal lifts, and deep plane lifts; these procedures may also have other names. The premise of the face-lifting is based on an understanding of the SMAS. The SMAS is continuous with the platysma inferiorly, although the platysma may have a more superior extent than realized. The SMAS is then manipulated, with or without the malar fat pad, in a superior lateral direction to lift and contour the face and neck. Although a rhytidectomy procedure is invasive, it offers more lasting benefits than thread lifts and fillers.

### Thread lift

Thread lifts have waxed and waned in popularity. Initially, thread lifts began with the use of permanent barbed sutures. Owing to high rates of extrusion, permanent sutures were replaced with intermediate lasting sutures made of polydioxanone (PDO).[35] A recent study found that 11.2% of patients had superficial displacement of the sutures, 6.2% had infection, and 6.2% had dimpling with results lasting about 6 months.[36] Newer, longer lasting sutures made of PLLA seem to offer an alternative material with increased potential. The ease of placement of PDO threads must be balanced with the limited duration and potential for skin reactivity and extrusion of the suture.[37,38]

## SOLUTIONS FOR THE AGING FACE BY AREA

When considering solutions to the aging face by area, it is important to remember that it is best to use combination of treatments (**Fig. 2**). Aging of the face is multifactorial and, therefore, sophisticated solutions to the face can lead to more comprehensive correction. Combination treatment involves understanding the root cause of excessive aging and treating each component as part of the palette of solutions. Finding a provider or a group of providers to help with each component can help patients to achieve a more satisfactory outcome.

### Brow and Forehead Area

Hairline recession is common for men and can be seen in a select group of women. Male pattern baldness has a typical pattern of temporal recession and elevation of the forehead, leading to a poorly framed face. Female hair loss is often more diverse and can be due to traction (ie, ponytails), hormonal changes, and a multitude of factors. For men, lowering the hairline often consists of the use of hair transplantation techniques. A variety of methods can be used, with the latest involving robotic transplantation. The overly long female forehead often involves a combination of surgical lowering and hair transplantation. Surgical lowering of the forehead is performed by first making an incision in front of the hairline in a pretrichial fashion. The scalp is then released along the galea and the pulled down to the desired area of the forehead. As much as 3 cm of skin is then excised and the hairline is then lowered. Further lowering to camouflage of the scar can be performed by using hair transplantation techniques.

Brow descent can cause excessive fullness along the eyelids and lead to a fatigued appearance. Contemporary brow-lifting techniques often focus on the use of endoscopes to release the brow's periosteum and suspend the periosteum cephalically. Less invasive techniques to lift the brow have become popular, such as the use of chemical brow lifts (botulinum toxin) as well as the use of suture suspension techniques. The use of PDO threads and PLLA threads have helped patients lift brows with minimal recovery time. PDO threads last approximately 6 months, whereas PLLA threads have a longevity of up to 18 months.

### Forehead and Temple Augmentation

The fat compartments of the temple as well as the brows lose volume over time. Placement of fillers or fat can help add to areas deficient in volume. Hyaluronic acid dermal fillers are the most commonly used fillers and may be injected into the desired area by trained personnel.

### Periorbital Area

The periorbital area consists of multiple different fat pads and muscular structures that act as slings and structural support for the overlying tissues. There is a global loss of volume around the orbit. In restoring a youthful periorbital appearance, popular approaches include injection of botulinum toxin, as well as placement of dermal hyaluronic acid fillers. For patients with excessive skin, termed dermatochalasis, skin can be removed by the use of an upper lid blepharoplasty. Removal of fat of the upper eyelid has become less popular in recent years owing to a better understanding of volume changes with age. Lower lid blepharoplasty involves remove of fat with or

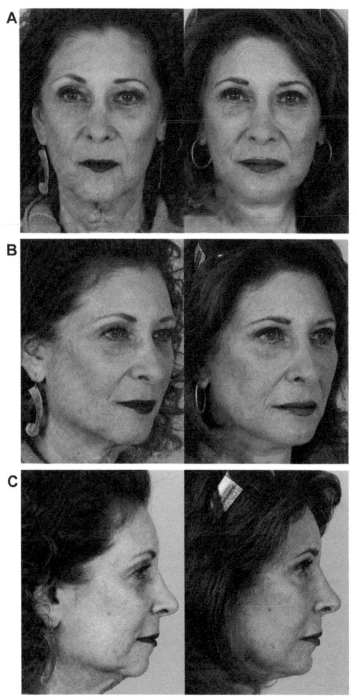

**Fig. 2.** (*A–C*) A combination of in-office and surgical procedures have provided this patient's face with a smooth and youthful appearance.

without skin tightening and/or removal. Periorbital fat from the lower eye area can be removed via an internal approach (transconjunctival) or external approach (subciliary). Volume can be added to the lower eye area with repositioning of fat, fat transfer from another area of the body, or the use of facial fillers. Skin tightening can be performed either via laser resurfacing, chemical peels, and/or physical removal of skin of the lower eyelid.

### Midface Area

The midface can be augmented in a variety of ways. Malar cheek fullness gives a youthful appearance and often augmentation of this region improves the appearance of the aging face. For augmentation, the malar cheek can be injected with hyaluronic acid dermal fillers or midface implants may be placed. Many of the newer fillers are specifically designed for midface augmentation, which includes Voluma (Allergan), Restylane Lift (Galderma), and Sculptra (Galderma). Although there are many facial filler products available, physicians should use discretion to choose products best for each patient's specific needs. The midface area can be lifted by itself with a combination of approaches, including midface lifts, deep plane facelifts, and thread lifts, as discussed. Midface lifts are performed via an endoscope and are typically involve a superior lateral suspension of the malar fat pad to the temple region. Deep plane facelifts involve lifting the malar fat pad and suspending it superiorly and laterally in conjunction with lifted skin and/or muscle. Thread lifts can be used as a minimally invasive lifting technique to suspend the face superiorly and include the use of either short acting sutures (PDO) or longer acting sutures (such as PLLA).

Rhytidectomy literally translates to the surgical removal of wrinkles or rhytides. In reality, most facelifts involve a combination of face lifting and neck lifting. This unified vision was first described in a paper describing the facial extent of the platysmal muscle by Drs. Rosenberg and Shah.[3] There are various types of rhytidectomy approaches, however the majority of these approaches involve elevating and lifting the SMAS to lift the face superiorly. Incisions are typically hidden behind the ear or along the hairline to avoid visible scars. Newer versions of lifts involve lifting and suspending the muscles and soft tissues of the face, which may result in a more natural appearance of the face.

### Nasal Area

Nasal lifting can be performed for the tip ptosis and internal nasal valve collapse experienced with aging. Patients may note the gradual appearance of dorsal humps, which can occur in part owing to a loss of support in the nasal tip. Minimally invasive approaches have been described, including placement of self-retaining anchoring sutures. More invasive approaches include performing lifting via an open or closed rhinoplasty, with a focus on the cartilaginous nasal tip. Major changes to the nose should be avoided in the aging patient owing to a strongly represented social identity.

### Chin Atrophy

Chin implantation may be used to augment the sunken appearance of the chin and prejowl region. These polymetric scaffolds allow for the chin to maintain a projected appearance over time and can often be inserted in a minimally invasive manner. Chin implants can be placed via an external or intraoral approach. Fillers can be used as an alternative but are often too soft to reliably restore a chin and create a large amount of projection.

### Excessive Fat in the Neck

Fat tends to accumulate in the lower part of the face and neck owing to gravitational descent as well as herniation through the separated platysmal bands. Removal of fat can be performed with a variety of techniques. Kybella is an injectable form of deoxycholic acid, a bile acid that causes destruction of fat cells, that has been used in a safe and effective manner to reduce submental fat.[39] It has been used off-label for injection into the jowl region. Liposuction can be safely performed in the neck area to contour and remove excessive fat. The removal of fat in older patients should be done in conjunction with skin removal (facelift) or use of radiofrequency device such as facetite/necktite to help prevent laxity of the neck skin. Radiofrequency-assisted liposuction has gained popularity in recent years and is an alternative to neck lifting for select patients wanting improvement in the neck without the periauricular scars of a facelift.

### Perioral Area

In the perioral region treatment options include botulinum toxin injections for selective muscular relaxation, adding volume to the lip area via filler application, and laser resurfacing. Perioral laser resurfacing improves rhytides through use of either the $CO_2$ laser or the erbium Nd:YAG laser previously described.

### Neck Bands

Noninvasive approaches to the improvement of neck bands are a popular option. Botulinum toxin may be injected into the platysmal bands to relax the muscles and lessen the appearance of both vertical and horizontal bands. Another nonsurgical approach includes the use of monopolar radiofrequency, which applies heat uniformly to the dermis at a controlled depth, leading to controlled scarring and contracture, giving the appearance of skin tightening. Fillers may also be injected into the skin to reduce the appearance of neck bands. Sculptra, an injectable and biodegradable substance composed of PLLA, is often used as a dermal filler. Injection of Sculptra into the skin can improve the appearance of thin and wrinkled, also known as crepey, skin. Surgically, the use of platysmaplasty in conjunction with a facelift can help decrease the appearance of neck bands. Typically, the bands of the platysma are imbricated together in a corset fashion. Some authors advocate the direct excision of platysmal bands.[40,41]

### Earlobes

Placement of dermal hyaluronic acid fillers into the earlobes has been described as a method of augmenting and enhancing the earlobes, which tend to become elongated and thin with age.

## REFERENCES

1. Gilhar A, Ullmann Y, Karry R, et al. Aging of human epidermis: reversal of aging changes correlates with reversal of keratinocyte fas expression and apoptosis. J Gerontol A Biol Sci Med Sci 2004;59(5):411–5.
2. Grove GL, Kligman AM. Age-associated changes in human epidermal cell renewal. J Gerontol 1983;38:137–42.
3. Cheng W, Yan-hua R, Fang-gang N, et al. The content and ratio of type I and III collagen in skin differ with age and injury. Afr J Biotechnol 2011;10(13):2524–9.
4. Heng JK, Aw DC, Tan KB. Solar elastosis in its papular form: uncommon, mistakable. Case Rep Dermatol 2014;6(1):124–8.

5. Zegarska B, Pietkun K, Giemza-Kucharska P, et al. Changes of Langerhans cells during skin ageing. Postepy Dermatol Alergol 2017;34(3):260–7.
6. Lambros V. Observations on periorbital and midface aging. Plast Reconstr Surg 2007;120:1367–76.
7. Kahn DM, Shaw RB. Overview of current thoughts on facial volume and aging. Facial Plast Surg 2010;26(5):350–5.
8. Truswell WH 4th. Aging changes of the periorbita, cheeks, and midface. Facial Plast Surg 2013;29(1):3–12.
9. Patterson CN. The aging nose: characteristics and correction. Otolaryngol Clin North Am 1980;13(2):275–88.
10. Garfein ES, Zide BM. Chin ptosis: classification, anatomy, and correction. Cranio-maxillofac Trauma Reconstr 2008;1(1):1–14.
11. Mendelson B, Wong CH. Changes in the facial skeleton with aging: implications and clinical applications in facial rejuvenation. Aesthetic Plast Surg 2012;36(4): 753–60.
12. Shah AR, Rosenberg D. Defining the facial extent of the platysma muscle. Arch Facial Plast Surg 2009;11(6):405–8.
13. Kostyuk V, Potapovich A, Albuhaydar AR, et al. Natural substances for prevention of skin photoaging: screening systems in the development of sunscreen and rejuvenation cosmetics. Rejuvenation Res 2018;21(2):91–101.
14. Addor FAS. Antioxidants in dermatology. An Bras Dermatol 2017;92(3):356–62.
15. Jurzak M, Latocha M, Gojniczek K, et al. Influence of retinoids on skin fibroblasts metabolism in vitro. Acta Pol Pharm 2008;65(1):85–91.
16. Brandhorst S, Choi IY, Wei M, et al. A periodic diet that mimics fasting promotes multi-system regeneration, enhanced cognitive performance, and healthspan. Cell Metab 2015;22(1):86–99.
17. Samaras N, Papadopoulou MA, Samaras D, et al. Off-label use of hormones as an antiaging strategy: a review. Clin Interv Aging 2014;9:1175–86. PMC. 25 Mar. 2018.
18. Wolff EF, Narayan D, Taylor HS. Long-term effects of hormone therapy on skin rigidity and wrinkles. Fertil Steril 2005;84(2):285–8.
19. Baulieu EE, Thomas G, Legrain S, et al. Dehydroepiandrosterone (DHEA), DHEA sulfate, and aging: contribution of the DHEAge study to a sociobiomedical issue. Proc Natl Acad Sci U S A 2000;97(8):4279–84.
20. Lephart ED. A review of the role of estrogen in dermal aging and facial attractiveness in women. J Cosmet Dermatol 2018;17(3):282–8.
21. Xiong BJ, Tan QW, Chen YJ, et al. The effects of platelet-rich plasma and adipose-derived stem cells on neovascularization and fat graft survival. Aesthetic Plast Surg 2018;42(1):1–8.
22. Saturveithan C, Premganesh G, Fakhrizzaki S, et al. Intra-articular hyaluronic acid (HA) and platelet rich plasma (PRP) injection versus hyaluronic acid (HA) injection alone in patients with grade III and IV knee osteoarthritis (OA): a retrospective study on functional outcome. Malays Orthop J 2016;10(2):35–40.
23. Preissig J, Hamilton K, Markus R. Current laser resurfacing technologies: a review that delves beneath the surface. Semin Plast Surg 2012;26(3):109–16.
24. Tanghetti EA. The histology of skin treated with a picosecond alexandrite laser and a fractional lens array. Lasers Surg Med 2016;48(7):646–52.
25. Bogdan Allemann I, Baumann L. Hyaluronic acid gel (Juvéderm™) preparations in the treatment of facial wrinkles and folds. Clin Interv Aging 2008;3(4):629–34.
26. Gogolewski S, Jovanovic M, Perren SM, et al. Tissue response and in vivo degradation of selected polyhydroxyacids: polylactides (PLA), poly(3-hydroxybutyrate)

(PHB), and poly(3-hydroxybutyrate-co-3-hydroxyvalerate) (PHB/VA). J Biomed Mater Res 1993;27(9):1135–48.

27. Lee JM, Kim YJ. Foreign body granulomas after the use of dermal fillers: pathophysiology, clinical appearance, histologic features, and treatment. Arch Plast Surg 2015;42(2):232.

28. Funt D, Pavicic T. Dermal fillers in aesthetics: an overview of adverse events and treatment approaches. Clin Cosmet Investig Dermatol 2013;6:295–316.

29. Dressler D, Saberi FA, Barbosa ER. Botulinum toxin: mechanisms of action. Arq Neuropsiquiatr 2005;63(1):180–5.

30. Codner MA, Kikkawa DO, Korn BS, et al. Blepharoplasty and brow lift. Plast Reconstr Surg 2010;126(1):1e–17e.

31. Rosenberg DB, Lattman J, Shah AR. Prevention of lower eyelid malposition after blepharoplasty: anatomic and technical considerations of the inside-out blepharoplasty. Arch Facial Plast Surg 2007;9(6):434–8.

32. Saban Y, Javier de B, Massa M. Nasal lift-nasal valve lift and nasal tip lift-preliminary results of a new technique using noninvasive self-retaining unidirectional nasal suspension with threads. Facial Plast Surg 2014;30(6):661–9.

33. Lee E. Aesthetic alteration of the chin. Semin Plast Surg 2013;27(3):155–60.

34. Schwarcz RM, Kotlus B. Complications of lower blepharoplasty and midface lifting. Clin Plast Surg 2015;42(1):63–71.

35. Karimi K, Reivitis A. Lifting the lower face with an absorbable polydioxanone (PDO) thread. J Drugs Dermatol 2017;16(9):932–4.

36. Suh DH, Jang HW, Lee SJ, et al. Outcomes of polydioxanone knotless thread lifting for facial rejuvenation. Dermatol Surg 2015;41(6):720–5.

37. Bertossi D, Botti G, Gualdi A, et al. Effectiveness, longevity, and complications of facelift by barbed suture insertion. Aesthet Surg J 2018. [Epub ahead of print].

38. Cobaleda Aristizabal AF, Sanders EJ, Barber FA. Adverse events associated with biodegradable lactide-containing suture anchors. Arthroscopy 2014;30(5):555–60.

39. Shamban AT. Noninvasive submental fat compartment treatment. Plast Reconstr Surg Glob Open 2016;4:e1155.

40. Mess SA. Lower face rejuvenation with injections: Botox, Juvederm, and Kybella for marionette lines and jowls. Plast Reconstr Surg Glob Open 2017;5(11):e1551.

41. Fogli AL. Skin and platysma muscle anchoring. Aesthetic Plast Surg 2008;32(3):531–41.

# Adult Head and Neck Health Care Needs for Individuals with Complex Chronic Conditions of Childhood

Sara Mixter, MD, MPH*, Rosalyn W. Stewart, MD, MBA, MS

## KEYWORDS

- Health care transition • Adults with chronic childhood conditions
- Youth with special health care needs • Adult head and neck health care

## KEY POINTS

- Millions of adults in the United states are currently living with what are termed chronic childhood conditions–childhood-onset conditions, about which adult providers often receive minimal training–and another half million youth with special health care needs enter adulthood each year and will undergo transition from pediatric to adult care.
- Many of these conditions have head and neck manifestations that can significantly affect communication and other tasks of daily living.
- Improved adult provider knowledge about these conditions can help maximize the health and functioning of patients with chronic conditions of childhood.

## INTRODUCTION

Approximately 18% of children in the United States have a chronic physical, emotional, behavioral, or developmental condition requiring more than usual medical care.[1] Advancements in medical and surgical care have led to well over 90% of these children with special health care needs surviving into adulthood.[2] Although family practice and internal medicine-pediatrics providers, and some subspecialists, may care for patients across the age spectrum, many of these children and their caretakers will be expected to transfer their primary and specialty care between pediatric and adult-focused medical providers as they age. This process has been termed health care transition.

In a position paper published in the journal *Pediatrics* in 1993, the Society for Adolescent Medicine defined health care transition as "the purposeful and planned movement of adolescents and young adults with chronic conditions from child-centered to adult-

Disclosure Statement: The authors have no relative disclosures.
Departments of Medicine and Pediatrics, Johns Hopkins University School of Medicine, 601 North Caroline Street, Suite 7143, Baltimore, MD 21287, USA
* Corresponding author.
*E-mail address:* smixter2@jhmi.edu

Med Clin N Am 102 (2018) 1055–1061
https://doi.org/10.1016/j.mcna.2018.06.007
0025-7125/18/© 2018 Elsevier Inc. All rights reserved.

medical.theclinics.com

centered care."[3] In the intervening years, multiple recommendations and consensus statements have delineated the steps necessary for patients, families, and providers to plan and navigate a successful transition.[4,5] However, there are significant barriers to transition between adult and pediatric care. One important barrier is discomfort on the part of adult providers in caring for youth with special health care needs because of lack of training in childhood-onset conditions.[6,7] This article reviews the otolaryngologic manifestations of chronic conditions of childhood of which adult providers may not be aware, as well as the basics of tracheostomy tube management. The intent is to increase awareness of potential head and neck complications in patients with select chronic conditions that extend across the lifespan.

## OTOLARYNGOLOGIC MANIFESTATIONS OF SELECTED CHRONIC CONDITIONS OF CHILDHOOD
### Autism Spectrum Disorder

Autism spectrum disorder (ASD) is a neurodevelopmental condition arising early in life and characterized by persistent deficits in social communication and interaction and restricted, repetitive patterns of interests, activities, or behaviors.[8] One in 68 US children has ASD, and prevalence has been shown to be steady with age, suggesting a similar rate among adults, even if less frequently diagnosed.[9] Hearing impairment is common in ASD, with mild-to-moderate hearing loss diagnosed in 7.9% and pronounced-to-profound hearing loss diagnosed in 3.5% of children and adolescents with autism in one study.[10] Hyperacusis was found in 18% of participants in the same study, and serous otitis media and associated conductive hearing loss were also significantly more common than typically developing controls. When an adult with ASD experiences a worsening in ability to communicate or other behavior change, it is important to consider new or worsening hearing loss as a potential etiology. There is also some evidence for higher rates of allergic rhinitis in patients with ASD, and that flares of allergic symptoms can contribute to behavior change.[11]

### Cerebral Palsy

The term cerebral palsy (CP) encompasses a diverse group of permanent motor disorders caused by injury to the fetal or infant brain.[12] CP occurs at a rate of 2 to 3 cases per 1000 infants born in the United States, and it is estimated that there are currently about 500,000 adults in the United States living with CP. Although CP itself is a motor disorder, it may be associated with other developmental problems, including intellectual disability, seizure disorder, and vision and hearing impairment. Hearing impairment can be congenital, but it may also worsen or develop over time, and adults with CP should be screened for hearing loss if symptoms or change in communication occur.[13] Sialorrhea occurs in about 40% of children and young people with CP. It can contribute to skin breakdown or aspiration (depending on whether is it anterior or posterior) and can be embarrassing for patients. Sialorrhea can be managed conservatively with speech therapy and behavioral strategies. Medications—particularly anticholinergics like glycopyrrolate and scopolamine—can also be used. More invasive strategies that would require comanagement with an otolaryngologist include botulinum toxin injections into the parotid and/or submandibular glands and surgical interventions.[14] The Sialorrhea Scoring Scale (SSS) is a 9-grade scale that has been used in individuals with developmental disabilities with excessive and bothersome sialorrhea.[15,16] The SSS ranges from 1 (least severe) to 9 (most severe) and can be used to track improvement in salivation with treatment.

### Down Syndrome

Also known as trisomy 21, Down syndrome occurs at a rate of 1 case per 700 live births to 1 case per 1000 live births.[17] It is associated with moderate-to-severe intellectual disability, as well as multiple other congenital anomalies, and it is the most common genetic cause of intellectual disability. About 90% of children born with Down syndrome will survive into adulthood, with median life expectancy in the 50s.[18] Morphologic abnormalities of the ear, nose, and throat are common among individuals with Down syndrome and give rise to referrals to otolaryngologists.[19] The abnormalities include shortened palate, macroglossia, and a narrow oropharynx and nasopharynx; these abnormalities, coupled with hypotonia—another characteristic feature of the syndrome—give rise to a high incidence of obstructive sleep apnea in individuals with Down syndrome.[20,21] Additionally, individuals with Down syndrome often have abnormalities in the paranasal sinuses, which coupled with delayed maturation of the immune system and ciliary dyskinesia, can contribute to a high incidence of chronic sinusitis.[22] About 50% of newborns with Down syndrome also have external ear canal stenosis; although this often improves with age, adults with Down Syndrome are particularly at risk for cerumen impaction, and may require otolaryngology referral for cleaning, sometimes even under anesthesia.[23] Hearing impairment is also common in children and adults with Down syndrome, and increases sharply after age 40; estimates are that between 51% and 74% of adults with Down syndrome have some degree of hearing loss.[24] Hearing screening is recommended every 2 years for adults with Down syndrome.[22,25]

### 22q11.2 Deletion Syndrome

22q11.2 deletion syndrome is estimated to occur at a rate of 1 case per 2000 live births, making it the most common microdeletion syndrome.[26] This blanket term includes multiple syndromes, including DiGeorge syndrome, conotruncal anomaly face syndrome, and velocardiofacial syndrome. Hearing loss is common, with estimates ranging between 40% and 75%, and it is thought to be multifactorial. Immune deficiency, palatal and eustachian tube dysfunction, and chronic middle ear effusions may all contribute, and a subset of patients may have congenital anomalies of the middle ear contributing to hearing loss.[27] Most patients will live into adulthood. Audiology assessment is recommended at the time of transition to adult primary care, and then as needed as apparent hearing issues arise.[26] In less than 5% of individuals with 22q11.2 deletion syndrome, subglottic stenosis, vocal cord paralysis, or laryngeal stenosis have been found and are associated with symptoms such as hoarseness, dyspnea, stridor, and cough.[27] Sequela associated with anatomic anomalies should be considered when progressive or new airway symptoms arise.

### Williams-Beuren Syndrome

Williams-Beuren syndrome, also known as Williams syndrome, is a rare neurogenetic developmental disorder characterized by typical facial features, which include dolichocephaly, asymmetry, bitemporal depressions, periorbital fullness, epicanthal folds, stellate irises, long philtrum, full lips, wide mouth, and dental malocclusion, which can contribute to significant dental caries.[28] It also is associated with mild-to-moderate intellectual disability and connective tissue abnormalities, which importantly can result in vascular obstructive disease.[29] Prevalence is estimated to be 1 case per 10,000 live births, and although lifespan is reduced, almost all children with Williams syndrome will live into adulthood.[30] Many persons with Williams-Beuren syndrome have hyperacusis and/or phonophobia, although this generally is less prevalent in adults than children. There is growing evidence that mild-to-moderate high-frequency hearing loss is common and progressive in adults with Williams-Beuren syndrome.[31] Baseline audiologic evaluation is recommended at age 30 to evaluate for sensorineural hearing loss, with follow-up evaluation at least every 5 years, or more frequently if there is evidence of hearing loss, until it stabilizes.[32] Adults with Williams-Beuren syndrome may also be more vulnerable to otitis media that typical adults. Persons with Williams-Beuren syndrome may also have significant cerumen build-up, and softening drops and cleanouts are recommended as needed.

### Tracheostomy Management

Patients transitioning from pediatric to adult care with a tracheostomy tube in place will require comanagement with an otolaryngologist, but it is important for primary care providers and generalists to know the basics of tracheostomy management to support patients and families, ensure there are appropriate supplies in the home for tracheostomy care, and help identify complications that may arise. Over the past few decades, the indications for pediatric tracheostomy have shifted from complications of acute infection to more chronic conditions, including allowing patients with chronic respiratory failure to be managed in the home setting.[33,34] Tracheostomy tubes are placed to allow for adequate ventilation, which may be mechanically assisted or nonassisted. One large category of conditions requiring tracheostomy for mechanical ventilation is neuromuscular diseases like muscular dystrophies or quadriplegia that cause ventilatory muscle weakness; once mechanical ventilation is started for these conditions it is generally needed life-long.[35] Underlying lung or airway disease, particularly bronchopulmonary dysplasia (lung disease associated with prematurity), may also cause chronic respiratory failure. Many of these conditions improve with age, and patients may be weaned off mechanical ventilation and decannulated by the time they transition to adult medicine; however, some cannot.[36]

Another major category of pediatric patients requiring tracheostomy placement — often without a requirement for ventilation — are those with airway obstruction, including congenital craniofacial anomaly syndromes and upper airway obstruction from conditions like subglottic stenosis or tracheomalacia.[36] Many of these children will see their obstruction improve as they grow, or may have surgeries as they get older to relieve obstruction, and be able to be decannulated, but some will continue to require tracheostomy at the time of transition to adult care.

There are several different types of tracheostomy tubes that may be encountered, and the type of tube is generally selected at the time of placement based on a variety of factors.[35] Tubes may be plastic, with an inner cannula that is removable for cleaning or replacement, and an outer cannula that stays in place, or metal. Tubes may also be cuffed or uncuffed. A cuffed tube has a circumferential balloon on the distal intratracheal segment that can be inflated to prevent leakage of air around the tube in patients who require mechanical ventilation. Patients who are breathing independently through their tracheostomy tube may have a speaking valve, a 1-way valve that attaches to the end of the tube and allows them to speak with their normal voice with the tracheostomy tube in place.[37] Many factors go into determining the schedule for tracheostomy tube change, but this is generally done every few weeks to months at home.[35] Routine tracheostomy care, which involves cleaning the area, changing the ties that secure the apparatus, and inner cannula cleaning, should occur daily, and caregivers are trained on this, appropriate use of suctioning, and emergency management at the time of placement.

There are several potential complications of tracheostomy of which the general provider should be aware. One is infection. It is not uncommon for a tracheostomy to become colonized with skin flora and typical upper respiratory flora, or other bacteria, so it is important to interpret tracheostomy cultures in light of this; culture results should be correlated with clinical presentation and the presence of other signs of infection, including fever, respiratory compromise, and significant white blood cells present in aspirates.[35] Obstruction can also occur. This can be acute (eg, from a mucus plug), and patients should travel with an extra tracheostomy tube in case obstruction occurs so the tube can be changed emergently. Chronic obstruction can also occur over time (eg, with the development of granulation tissue or stenosis).[37] Another rare but serious set of complications are fistulae, including tracheocutaneous fistula, tracheoesophageal fistula, or vascular fistulas, including innominate artery fistula (although this generally occurs in the first few weeks after tracheostomy placement).[35,37]

## SUMMARY

There are already millions of adults living with chronic childhood conditions in the United States, and every year another 500,000 youth with special health care needs enter adulthood.[2] The transition from pediatric to adult care is a complex process, and increasing adult provider knowledge of the conditions and needs of these individuals is an important piece of the puzzle. The otolaryngologic manifestations reviewed here have serious potential implications for patients, from limiting their ability to communicate effectively, to increasing their risk for serious infections. By becoming familiar with the conditions commonly encountered in these patients, especially their potential complications and associated screening recommendations, adult providers can help maximize the health and functioning of their patients with chronic conditions of childhood.

## REFERENCES

1. Newacheck PW, Strickland B, Shonkoff JP, et al. An epidemiologic profile of children with special health care needs. Pediatrics 1998;102(1 Pt 1):117–23.
2. A consensus statement on health care transitions for young adults with special health care needs. Pediatrics 2002;110(6 Pt 2):1304–6.
3. Blum RW, Garell D, Hodgman CH, et al. Transition from child-centered to adult health-care systems for adolescents with chronic conditions. A position paper of the society for adolescent medicine. J Adolesc Health 1993;14(7):570–6.
4. Transition of care provided for adolescents with special health care needs. American Academy of Pediatrics committee on children with disabilities and committee on adolescence. Pediatrics 1996;98(6 Pt 1):1203–6.
5. Cooley WC, Sagerman PJ. Supporting the health care transition from adolescence to adulthood in the medical home. Pediatrics 2011;128(1):182–200.
6. Peter NG, Forke CM, Ginsburg KR, et al. Transition from pediatric to adult care: Internists' perspectives. Pediatrics 2009;123(2):417–23.
7. Callahan ST, Winitzer RF, Keenan P. Transition from pediatric to adult-oriented health care: a challenge for patients with chronic disease. Curr Opin Pediatr 2001;13(4):310–6.
8. American Psychiatric Association. Diagnostic and statistical manual of mental disorders. 5th edition. Arlington (VA): American Psychiatric Association; 2013.
9. Christensen DL. Prevalence and characteristics of autism spectrum disorder among children aged 8 years—Autism and developmental disabilities monitoring network, 11 sites, United States, 2012. MMWR Surveill Summ 2016;65:1–23. Available at: https://www.cdc.gov/mmwr/volumes/65/ss/ss6503a1.htm.

10. Rosenhall U, Nordin V, Sandström M, et al. Autism and hearing loss. J Autism Dev Disord 1999;29(5):349–57.
11. Miyazaki C, Koyama M, Ota E, et al. Allergies in children with autism spectrum disorder: a systematic review and meta-analysis. Rev J Autism Dev Disord 2015;2(4):374–401.
12. Colver A, Fairhurst C, Pharoah POD. Cerebral palsy. Lancet 2014;383(9924): 1240–9.
13. Peterson H, Lenski M, Cooley J, et al. Cerebral palsy and aging. Dev Med Child Neurol 2009;51:16–23.
14. Glader L, Delsing C, Hughes A, et al. Care pathways: sialorrhea. Milwaukee (WI): American Academy for Cerebral Palsy and Developmental Medicine; 2016.
15. Arbouw MEL, Movig KLL, Koopmann M, et al. Glycopyrrolate for sialorrhea in Parkinson disease: a randomized, double-blind, crossover trial. Neurology 2010; 74(15):1203–7.
16. Mier RJ, Bachrach SJ, Lakin RC, et al. Treatment of sialorrhea with glycopyrrolate: a double-blind, dose-ranging study. Arch Pediatr Adolesc Med 2000;154(12): 1214–8.
17. Parker SE, Mai CT, Canfield MA, et al. Updated national birth prevalence estimates for selected birth defects in the United States, 2004-2006. Birth Defects Res A Clin Mol Teratol 2010;88(12):1008–16.
18. Presson AP, Partyka G, Jensen KM, et al. Current estimate of Down syndrome population prevalence in the United States. J Pediatr 2013;163(4):1163–8.
19. Mitchell RB, Ellen C, James K. Ear, nose and throat disorders in children with Down syndrome. Laryngoscope 2009;113(2):259–63.
20. Marcus CL, Keens TG, Bautista DB, et al. Obstructive sleep apnea in children with Down syndrome. Pediatrics 1991;88(1):132–9.
21. Kanamori G, Witter M, Brown J, et al. Otolaryngologic manifestations of Down syndrome. Otolaryngol Clin North Am 2000;33(6):1285–92.
22. Rodman R, Pine HS. The otolaryngologist's approach to the patient with Down syndrome. Otolaryngol Clin North Am 2012;45(3):viii.
23. Shott SR. Down syndrome: common otolaryngologic manifestations. Am J Med Genet 2006;142C(3):131–40.
24. Keiser H, Montague J, Wold D, et al. Hearing loss of Down syndrome adults. Am J Ment Defic 1981;85(5):467–72.
25. Jensen KM, Bulova PD. Managing the care of adults with down's syndrome. BMJ 2014;349:g5596.
26. Fung WL, Butcher NJ, Costain G, et al. Practical guidelines for managing adults with 22q11.2 deletion syndrome. Genet Med 2015;17(8):599–609.
27. Dyce O, McDonald-McGinn D, Kirschner RE, et al. Otolaryngologic manifestations of the 22q11.2 deletion syndrome. Arch Otolaryngol Head Neck Surg 2002;128(12):1408–12.
28. Morris CA, Demsey SA, Leonard CO, et al. Natural history of Williams syndrome: physical characteristics. J Pediatr 1988;113(2):318–26.
29. Williams syndrome - NORD (national organization for rare disorders). NORD (National Organization for Rare Disorders) Web site. 2006. Available at: https://rarediseases.org/rare-diseases/williams-syndrome/. Accessed April 4, 2018.
30. Pober BR. Williams–Beuren syndrome. N Engl J Med 2010;362(3):239–52.
31. Marler JA, Sitcovsky JL, Mervis CB, et al. Auditory function and hearing loss in children and adults with Williams syndrome: cochlear impairment in individuals with otherwise normal hearing. Am J Med Genet 2010;154C(2):249–65.

32. Pober BR, Morris CA. Diagnosis and management of medical problems in adults with Williams–Beuren syndrome. Am J Med Genet 2007;145C(3):280–90.
33. Lawrason A, Kavanagh K. Pediatric tracheotomy: are the indications changing? Int J Pediatr Otorhinolaryngol 2013;77(6):922–5.
34. Gergin O, Adil EA, Kawai K, et al. Indications of pediatric tracheostomy over the last 30 years: has anything changed? Int J Pediatr Otorhinolaryngol 2016;87: 144–7.
35. Barto TL. Respiratory care of adults with chronic pulmonary disease. In: Pilapil M, DeLaet DE, Kuo AA, et al, editors. Care of adults with chronic childhood conditions. Alexandria (VA): Society of General Internal Medicine; 2016. p. 303–8.
36. McPherson ML, Shekerdemian L, Goldsworthy M, et al. A decade of pediatric tracheostomies: Indications, outcomes, and long-term prognosis. Pediatr Pulmonol 2017;52(7):946–53.
37. Heffner JE, Hess D. Tracheostomy management in the chronically ventilated patient. Clin Chest Med 2001;22(1):55–69.

# Chronic Ear Disease

Susan D. Emmett, MD, MPH[a],*, John Kokesh, MD[b], David Kaylie, MD[c]

## KEYWORDS

- Eustachian tube dysfunction • Otitis media • Cholesteatoma • Hearing loss

## KEY POINTS

- Chronic ear disease is common in primary care settings.
- Presentation can range from asymptomatic findings on physical examination to critically ill patients with intracranial complications.
- Internists represent the first line in diagnosis of these conditions, making partnership between internal medicine and otolaryngology essential.

## INTRODUCTION

Chronic ear disease is composed of a spectrum of otologic disorders that frequently present to primary care providers. Otitis media has long been acknowledged as one of the most common diagnoses in primary care settings worldwide.[1] Chronic suppurative otitis media, which results from an episode of acute otitis that has evolved into persistent otorrhea, is estimated to affect 65 to 330 million individuals globally.[2] Both developed and developing countries are affected by chronic ear disease, with certain populations known to be at particularly high risk, including Alaska Native and Indigenous populations of Canada and Greenland, Native Americans, Australian Aborigines, and New Zealand Maori and other South Pacific Island populations.[2,3]

Eustachian tube dysfunction (ETD) is thought to be the underlying pathology resulting in the spectrum of chronic ear disease.[4,5] ETD and otitis media have been extensively studied in children; however, recent epidemiologic data suggest that these conditions warrant attention in adults. Vila and colleagues[6] observed in an analysis of the National Ambulatory Medical Care Survey and National Hospital Ambulatory Medical Care Survey that outpatient visits related to ETD, otitis media with effusion, and tympanic membrane retraction exceeded 2 million per year in both the 0 to 20-year age group and among patients older than 20 years. The prevalence of visits

Disclosure Statement: The authors have nothing to disclose.
[a] Head and Neck Surgery and Communication Sciences, Duke University School of Medicine, Duke Global Health Institute, DUMC Box 3805, Durham, NC 27710, USA; [b] Department of Otolaryngology, Alaska Native Medical Center, 4315 Diplomacy Drive, Anchorage, AK 99508, USA; [c] Head and Neck Surgery and Communication Sciences, Duke University School of Medicine, DUMC Box 3805, Durham, NC 27710, USA
* Corresponding author.
E-mail address: susan.emmett@duke.edu

in adults in that study was 77% of the prevalence in children. Hearing loss frequently accompanies chronic ear disease due to disruption of the ossicles and/or tympanic membrane. When left untreated, grave intratemporal and intracranial complications can ensue. We have described the pathophysiology and presenting symptoms of the spectrum of chronic ear disease disorders, along with complications, to assist in identification of these patients in the primary care setting. Although much of the management of chronic ear disease is surgical, initial presentation of these patients in primary care makes partnership between internists and otolaryngologists essential.

## PATIENT HISTORY

The presentation of patients with chronic ear disease ranges from asymptomatic findings on physical examination to critically ill patients with intracranial complications. Common patient complaints include aural fullness, hearing loss, and intermittent otorrhea. Otalgia, or ear pain, as well as an inability to clear the ears, may also be described. It is important to determine whether the patient has experienced vertigo, including the timing of vertigo symptoms in relation to any ear complaints. Patients should be questioned about a history of ear infections, particularly in childhood, and whether they have undergone any ear surgeries. Concomitant allergic rhinitis, rhinosinusitis, reflux, and smoke exposure should be elucidated.[7,8] Common presenting symptoms are described with each classification of chronic ear disease in the next section.

## PATHOPHYSIOLOGY
### Normal Anatomy

Understanding the pathophysiology of chronic ear disease begins with the normal anatomy of the temporal bone. The temporal bone contains the body's hearing and balance functions. The inner ear is composed of the cochlea and vestibular systems. The tympanic cavity is an air-filled middle ear cleft that contains the ossicular chain (hearing bones) and is bordered laterally by the tympanic membrane (**Fig. 1**). The facial nerve, chorda tympani nerve, and Jacobson nerve (tympanic branch of the

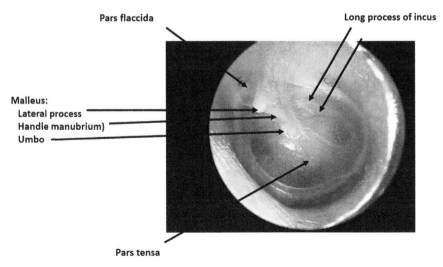

**Fig. 1.** Otoscopic view of a normal left tympanic membrane.

glossopharyngeal) run through this space. The mastoid air cell system exists in continuity with the tympanic cavity and contributes to mucosal gas exchange and regulation of pressure within the middle ear cleft.

The tympanic cavity is connected to the nasopharynx by the Eustachian tube, a complex, dynamic canal of mucosa, cartilage, muscles, and bone that allows gas exchange between the nasopharynx and middle ear. Normal gas exchange through the Eustachian tube maintains pressure in the middle ear cleft that is equivalent to atmospheric pressure (760 mm Hg), which enables optimal sound transmission.[9] The size of the mastoid air cells affects compliance of this system.

The tympanic membrane is composed of the pars tensa and pars flaccida. The pars tensa contains 3 cell layers, from squamous epithelium laterally to a middle fibrous layer and medial mucosal layer that is contiguous with the mucosal lining of the middle ear cleft. The fibrous layer is absent in pars flaccida, and cilia are absent on the medial mucosal lining of this portion of the tympanic membrane.[10]

## Eustachian Tube Dysfunction

The Eustachian tube plays a central role in chronic ear disease, with ETD noted in up to 70% of patients undergoing middle ear surgery.[11] ETD impairs pressure equilibration in the middle ear and can lead to perturbations in middle ear aeration. Resulting symptoms include aural fullness, hearing loss, otalgia, and autophony, which is hearing your own voice loudly in one or both ears.

There are 2 categories of ETD: dilatory and patulous. Dilatory dysfunction is most commonly caused by mucosal inflammation, which impairs the dilatory function of the Eustachian tube. Contributing factors include allergic rhinitis, chronic rhinosinusitis, reflux, smoke exposure, genetics, and underlying conditions, such as cleft palate.[7,8] The hallmark of patulous ETD is positional autophony of voice and interior body sounds, such as breathing, which improve when lying supine. Patulous ETD is treated differently from obstructive pathology, with a focus on augmentation or reconstructive procedures.[12]

When evaluating a patient with aural fullness, there are other etiologies besides ETD dysfunction that should be considered, including temporomandibular joint disorders, superior semicircular canal dehiscence syndrome, Meniere disease, and elevated intracranial pressure.

## Classifications of Chronic Ear Disease

There are multiple manifestations of chronic ear disease that exist on a pathologic spectrum intrinsically tied to ETD. Sustained negative pressure in the middle ear leads to the formation of an inflammatory exudate or effusion. Repeated episodes of negative pressure contribute to the pathology of tympanic membrane retraction, including retraction pockets, atelectasis, adhesive otitis media, and cholesteatoma. The mastoid cavity is also important in regulating gas exchange in the tympanic cavity. Chronic ETD in early childhood often results in a sclerotic or small mastoid in an adult, which is more vulnerable to pressure changes and increasingly likely to result in middle ear pathology.[9]

### Otitis media

Otitis media is classified by timing of symptoms and presence of inflammation. Acute otitis media (AOM) represents inflammation of the middle ear with acute onset and rapid resolution (**Fig. 2**). AOM is often associated with fever and otalgia. There should also be hearing loss because the middle ear is filled with infected fluid, impairing tympanic membrane and ossicular movement. Otitis media with effusion (OME), on the

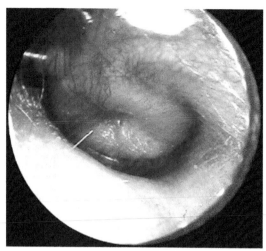

**Fig. 2.** AOM. There is purulent fluid behind an intact tympanic membrane and prominent vasculature.

other hand, consists of fluid in the middle ear space with no obvious signs of inflammation (**Fig. 3**). This can be found after an infection resolves in which the fluid is sterile. An acute effusion lasts less than 3 weeks, subacute from 3 weeks to 3 months, and chronic for more than 3 months.[1] The effusion seen after an AOM can take several weeks to resolve after the infection is gone. This requires patience to let the effusion resolve on its own.

Adults with chronic OME will often complain of fullness in the ear and will have a conductive hearing loss. In patients with unilateral OME, it is important to rule out nasopharyngeal pathology.

### Tympanic membrane perforations
Perforations are characterized by a variety of descriptions without a single unifying classification scheme. They can be described based on location (central vs marginal),

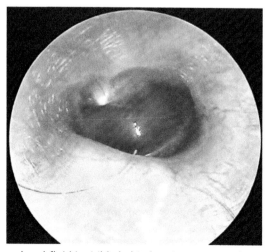

**Fig. 3.** OME. Straw-colored fluid is visible behind an intact tympanic membrane.

size (eg, subtotal), or chronicity (acute or chronic). Acute perforations are often secondary to AOM or trauma. Perforations secondary to infection are usually small and generally heal spontaneously, although ongoing infection may lead to a chronic perforation.[13] The inciting inflammation may resolve, resulting in a dry perforation (**Fig. 4**), or there can be ongoing infection, which is characterized by otorrhea (**Fig. 5**). Traumatic perforations can result from penetrating or blunt trauma, barotrauma, or acoustic trauma. Perforations secondary to water sports, heat, corrosives, and lightning are least likely to heal spontaneously.[14] Nonhealing perforations should be referred to an otolaryngologist for surgical management.

### Chronic suppurative otitis media

When drainage from a tympanic membrane perforation continues for more than 3 months, it is described as chronic suppurative otitis media (CSOM) (**Fig. 6**). Patients with CSOM may enter quiescent periods without otorrhea or experience intermittent drainage. CSOM can be associated with cholesteatoma. All patients with CSOM require management by an otolaryngologist, and many require surgery. Hearing outcomes vary depending on severity of disease and ossicular erosion.

### Tympanic membrane collapse: retraction, atelectasis, and adhesive otitis media

There is a broad spectrum of tympanic membrane collapse, ranging from mild retraction (**Fig. 7**) to adhesive otitis media affecting the entire tympanic membrane (**Fig. 8**). Similar to OME, adhesive otitis media is theorized to develop due to sustained negative pressure in the middle ear from ETD, in combination with epithelial proliferation secondary to chronic inflammation.[15] There are several classification schemes for retraction pockets that are intended to guide surgical decision making and predict hearing outcomes.[16–18] Retraction pockets may develop in pars flaccida (**Fig. 9**) or pars tensa (**Fig. 10**). Deep pockets where the base cannot be visualized, as well as retraction pockets with debris, are concerning for cholesteatoma formation and generally require surgical management. Atelectasis of the tympanic membrane and adhesive otitis media can damage the ossicles over time secondary to erosion (**Fig. 11**). These patients are followed carefully by otolaryngologists and often require interventions ranging from tympanostomy tube placement to tympanoplasty, ossicular chain reconstruction, or tympanomastoidectomy. Of note, internists may discover

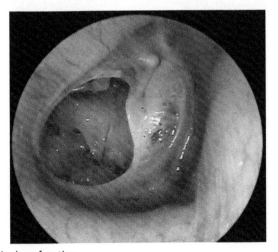

**Fig. 4.** Dry, marginal perforation.

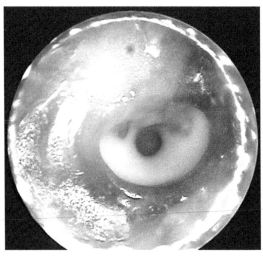

**Fig. 5.** Central perforation with otorrhea.

a deep retraction pocket on routine physical examination without related complaints from the patient.[19] These patients should be asked about hearing loss, fullness, otalgia, and prior infections and referred to an otolaryngologist for monitoring and further management.

### Cholesteatoma

Cholesteatoma is a collection of epithelial cells in the middle ear that is present in an estimated 40% of cases of CSOM.[20,21] Cholesteatoma can be congenital, believed to develop from embryonic cell nests, or acquired, which is far more common.[22,23] Acquired cholesteatomas originate from the epithelium of the tympanic membrane. There are 3 primary theories to explain acquired cholesteatoma formation. The

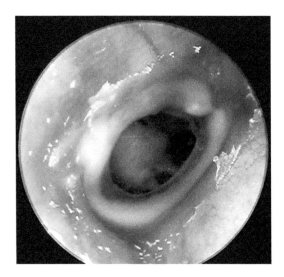

**Fig. 6.** CSOM.

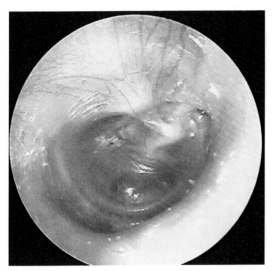

**Fig. 7.** Mild tympanic membrane retraction.

retraction pocket theory posits that retraction secondary to negative pressure from ETD traps squamous debris, leading to formation of a cholesteatoma sac. The proliferation theory suggests that chronic inflammation stimulates growth of the basal cells in the stratum corneum layer of pars flaccida, leading a disruption of self-cleaning and resulting cholesteatoma formation. Lastly, the migration theory suggests cholesteatomas form from epithelial migration through an existing perforation.[24] In reality, each of these theories likely plays a role in etiology, as cholesteatomas can arise from retraction pockets in pars flaccida or pars tensa, as well as from chronic perforations.

Warning signs of cholesteatoma include deep retraction pockets (**Fig. 12**), keratin debris that cannot be fully removed during office examination (**Fig. 13**), and chronic

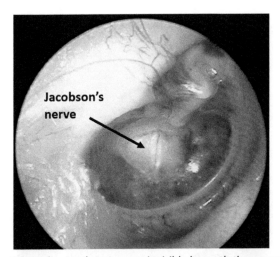

**Fig. 8.** Adhesive otitis media. Jacobson's nerve is visible beneath the severely retracted tympanic membrane.

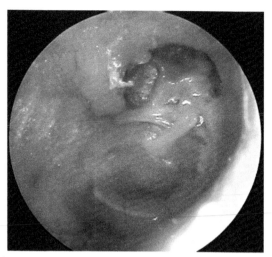

Fig. 9. Pars flaccida retraction pocket.

otorrhea. Cholesteatoma is locally destructive, eroding bone through absorptive oste-itis (**Fig. 14**). It is managed surgically, and any suspicion of a cholesteatoma warrants referral.

## PHYSICAL EXAMINATION

A thorough otoscopic examination is essential when evaluating patients for chronic ear disease. Binocular microscopy provides a 3-dimensional view of the tympanic membranes and is the diagnostic tool of choice for otoscopic examination. Often a microscope is not available within primary care offices, however, in which case a hand-held otoscope must suffice. A complete examination evaluates the skin of the external auditory canal, tympanic membrane, visible portions of the ossicular chain, and

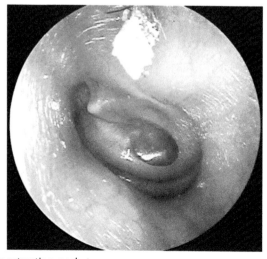

Fig. 10. Pars tensa retraction pocket.

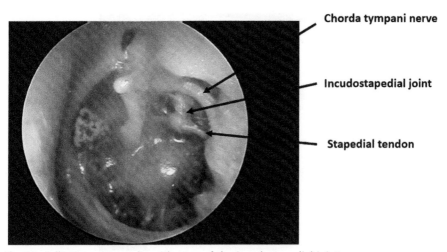

**Chorda tympani nerve**

**Incudostapedial joint**

**Stapedial tendon**

**Fig. 11.** Adhesive otitis media with pexy of the incudostapedial joint.

middle ear space. Pneumatic otoscopy is a helpful adjunct to assess tympanic membrane mobility, as is asking the patient to "pop their ears" by Valsalva during the examination.

In addition to otoscopic examination, tuning forks are used to assess hearing and determine the nature of a patient's hearing loss. The Weber test is performed by placing a vibrating 512 Hz tuning fork midline on a patient's forehead or bony dorsum of the nose and asking whether the patient hears the sound on the right, left, or middle. The anterior incisors also can be used if the patient does not hear the tuning fork from other locations. The Weber test will lateralize to the better-hearing ear in patients with sensorineural hearing loss and to the worse hearing ear in conductive hearing loss. Lateralization occurs with even 5 dB of conductive hearing loss.[25] If hearing is normal, or if the patient's hearing loss is symmetric, the Weber test will be midline. With the Rinne test, a patient is asked to

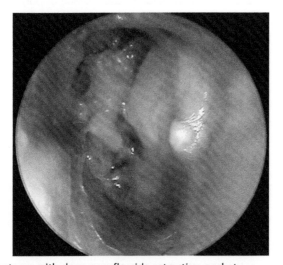

**Fig. 12.** Cholesteatoma with deep pars flaccida retraction pocket.

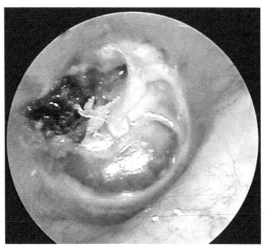

**Fig. 13.** Keratin debris suggesting underlying cholesteatoma.

listen to a tuning fork vibrating in the air near the auricle and postauricularly against the mastoid bone. If bone conduction is louder than air, this is described as reversing forks and indicates a conductive hearing loss. A patient who reverses the Rinne with a 512-Hz fork has a 15 to 20 dB hearing loss, and reversal with a 1024 Hz fork suggests at least a 30-dB loss.[25] The Rinne test should be performed bilaterally.

Lastly, physical examination of patients with chronic ear disease should include an assessment of the facial nerve and palpation of the temporomandibular joints. In the otolaryngologist's office, these patients are also evaluated for nasopharyngeal pathology by using nasopharyngoscopy.

## CLINICAL FINDINGS
### Otoscopy

Otoscopic examination may reveal changes in the external auditory canal, including edema, granulation tissue, or otorrhea. Granulation tissue or polyps in the ear canal

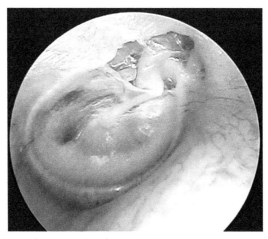

**Fig. 14.** Cholesteatoma demonstrating bony erosion.

are concerning for underlying pathology, such as cholesteatoma. The tympanic membrane may demonstrate a dry perforation, or in cases of ongoing infection, a perforation with otorrhea. ETD presents with a range of pathologic findings described in the pathophysiology section, including retraction pockets, atelectasis, adhesive otitis media, and OME. Care should be taken during the examination to note ossicular erosion, tympanosclerosis (scarring), and keratin debris.

## Microbiology

Pathogens involved in chronic ear disease vary based on chronicity of the infection. In AOM, the most common organisms are *Haemophilus influenzae* (non-typeable), *Streptococcus pneumoniae,* and *Moraxella catarrhalis*.[26] Viruses often contribute to preceding upper respiratory tract infections and lead to mucosal edema but are not considered causative.[27] The most common organisms in CSOM, by contrast, are *Pseudomonas aeruginosa,* methicillin-resistant *Staphylococcus aureus*, methicillin-sensitive *S aureus,* and coagulase-negative *Staphylococci*.[28,29] Anaerobic bacteria, which act synergistically with *S aureus and P aeruginosa,* are cultured in 50% of chronically draining ears.[30] Common anaerobes include *Peptostreptococcus* spp, *Bacteroides fragilis, Fusobacterium* spp, *Prevotella* spp, *and Porphyromonas* spp.[30] The microbiology of CSOM appears to be changing over time, with CSOM secondary to community-acquired methicillin-resistant *S aureus* increasing from 0.7% to 11.4% from 1998 to 2006.[31] There is also geographic variation in CSOM pathogens. In Nigeria, for example, *Klebsiella, Escherichia coli,* and *Streptococcus* were the most commonly cultured bacteria in CSOM.[32] Fungi are responsible for an estimated 5% of CSOM cases and include *Aspergillus* spp and *Candida* spp.[29,33] CSOM secondary to tuberculosis is rare, estimated at fewer than 1% of cases.[34]

There is growing evidence of biofilms in CSOM, both in cases with and without cholesteatoma.[35–39] Biofilms resist antibiotics through multiple mechanisms, including harboring metabolically inactive cells that can repopulate if active cells are killed by antibiotics, as well as producing an extracellular polymeric substance that shields the biofilm.[40] Treatment of a recalcitrant CSOM infection in which biofilms have been implicated often requires both physical removal of the biofilm and antibiotic therapy. There are, however, some topical medications commonly used by otolaryngologists, such as gentian violet, that have been shown to inhibit biofilm formation in vitro.[41]

In the era of increasing antibiotic resistance, it is important to note that topically administered antibiotics are vastly preferred over systemic therapy for chronic ear disease. The drug concentrations achieved with topical administration are many orders of magnitude higher than systemically delivered doses. Topical therapy is often effective even when standard cultures show resistance because the concentrations are so much higher than those used for resistance testing in microbiology laboratories. Ototoxicity is a concern when high drug concentrations are locally delivered to the middle ear space. Potentially ototoxic preparations are avoided when a perforation is present, with quinolone-based drops preferred when the tympanic membrane is not intact.

## IMAGING AND ADDITIONAL TESTING

A thorough history and otoscopic examination of the ear are the 2 most important diagnostic tools for chronic ear disease. Once a patient is referred, an audiometric evaluation is performed that includes air and bone conduction pure tone audiometry, as well as tympanometry. Audiometry delineates the type and severity of hearing loss.

Tympanometry assesses middle ear pressure and is helpful in confirming cases of retraction, effusion, and perforation. These patients have mild to severe conductive hearing loss and may present with a mixed loss if age-related hearing loss is also present. The severity of conductive hearing loss does not directly correlate with severity of chronic ear disease.[19]

Nasopharyngoscopy is performed to evaluate for nasopharyngeal pathology in cases of ETD. Imaging with high-resolution computed tomography (CT) of the temporal bone is used in cases suspicious for cholesteatoma or when complications of chronic ear disease are present.

## DIAGNOSTIC DILEMMAS
### Tuberculous Otitis

Accounting for less than 1% of chronic otitis and presenting with variable symptoms, tuberculous otitis can be difficult to diagnosis. It is nevertheless important to differentiate this etiology of chronic ear disease because an anti-tuberculosis regimen is a fundamental aspect of treatment. Patients most commonly present with otorrhea. Tympanic membrane perforations are also frequent in tuberculous otitis, and other presenting symptoms may include hearing loss, otalgia, tinnitus, vertigo, and facial palsy.[42] Diagnosis is most reliably obtained from tissue biopsy during surgery.

### Complications of Otitis Media

Before antibiotics became widely available in the 1940s, life-threatening complications of otitis media were common. The prevalence of complications has plummeted over the past 80 years, allowing a shift from treating grave complications in patients with chronic ear disease to focusing on long-term management and hearing restoration. Yet despite the improvements associated with antibiotic management, complications of otitis continue to arise in both developing *and* developed countries.[43] As we move into an era in which compromised immunity from aging of the population, diabetes mellitus, and immunosuppressive drugs may further open the door to opportunistic infections, it is essential to understand the telling signs and symptoms to avoid dangerous delays in treatment. Although management is often surgical, internal medicine represents the first line in diagnosis of these critically ill patients.

Intratemporal and intracranial complications can result from both acute and chronic otitis media, with chronic otitis media representing the source in 80% of cases in a recent Brazilian study by Penido and colleagues.[43] Spread of the infection can occur through 3 routes, including hematogenous spread, thrombophlebitis, and direct extension through congenital or acquired bony defects.[44,45]

### Intratemporal complications

*Acute mastoiditis* evolves from otitis media when the antrum connecting the middle ear and mastoid is blocked by granulation tissue and inflammation, leading to a walled-off collection in the mastoid. This presents with breakdown of the bony trabeculae of the mastoid, often deemed coalescent mastoiditis by radiology, and presents with a protruding ear and erythematous, tender mastoid. Therapy includes empiric antibiotic therapy, myringotomy, and cortical mastoidectomy in patients who do not respond to medical treatment. It is important to note that any imaging of a patient with otitis media will show opacified air cells in the mastoid; however, opacification is not clinically mastoiditis. True mastoiditis has bony destruction and loss of septations. *Petrous apicitis*, an infection of the petrous apex portion of the temporal bone, presents with the Gradenigo triad of otorrhea, retro-orbital pain, and abducens palsy. This constellation of symptoms is secondary to the anatomy of the petrous apex, with trigeminal irritation causing retro-orbital pain and abducens palsy due to compression of the Dorello canal. MRI with gadolinium is used for diagnosis, along with temporal bone CT to assess the petrous air cells. The characteristic imaging findings are heterogeneity on T1 postcontrast images, with hyperintensity on T2 and loss of petrous apex bony septations on CT. Treatment consists of empiric antibiotic therapy and surgical drainage.

*Labyrinthine fistula* develops in approximately 10% of cholesteatomas and is second only to erosion of the ossicular chain in frequency of intratemporal complications of chronic ear disease.[46,47] Both a history of imbalance in a patient with chronic ear disease and nystagmus from pressure changes in the external auditory canal (fistula test) raise suspicion for fistula. Temporal bone CT can assist in diagnosis and operative planning for management. *Labyrinthitis* may develop from direct bacterial spread to the labyrinth or from diffusion of inflammatory mediators across the round window membrane or labyrinthine fistula.[48] Symptoms include severe vertigo, sensorineural hearing loss, and tinnitus. On physical examination, spontaneous nystagmus toward the affected side is present initially but transitions to nystagmus away from the affected side as the labyrinthine function declines over the ensuing 24 to 48 hours. It is important to note that the labyrinth communicates with the subarachnoid space, so labyrinthitis can progress to ascending meningitis. Both CT and MRI are used in the workup, with CT revealing predisposing conditions such as a Mondini malformation or labyrinthine fistula, and MRI demonstrating hyperintensity on T1 postcontrast images and increased fluid-attenuated inversion recovery signal intensity in the labyrinth. Treatment consists of high-dose steroids and antibiotics with cerebrospinal fluid (CSF) penetration. There should be a low threshold to perform a lumbar puncture if meningeal symptoms such as headache, nuchal rigidity, or mental status changes develop.

*Facial paralysis* can develop from otitis media. Exact mechanisms are unknown but are theorized to be secondary to direct spread of infection in areas of dehiscence of the Fallopian canal or neural edema evolving from nearby infection and inflammation, leading to ischemia. A temporal bone CT is obtained, and the patient is treated with empiric antibiotics, steroids, and myringotomy with tube placement.[49] Cortical mastoidectomy is considered in patients who do not respond to medical management. Lastly, *temporal bone encephalocele* and *CSF leak* can develop in the setting of chronic ear disease. Patients may present with conductive hearing loss and otorrhea. When clear otorrhea is suspicious for CSF, a specimen for beta-2 transferrin should be collected and thin-section CT of the skull base obtained. Resolution with conservative management tends to be low in patients with chronic ear disease, making early surgical repair preferable.[50,51]

### Intracranial complications

*Otogenic meningitis* is the most common intracranial complication of otitis media and is more likely to occur in settings of acute, suppurative infection.[44,52–54] Patients present with typical meningeal symptoms, such as headache, photophobia, nuchal rigidity, and altered mental status. CT of the temporal bone and lumbar puncture should be performed during the diagnostic workup. Treatment consists of intravenous (IV) antibiotics with CSF penetration, with the addition of steroids having been shown to reduce neurologic sequelae.[55] Otorrhea will generally be present if a tympanic membrane perforation has already occurred. If the tympanic membrane is intact, myringotomy and tympanostomy tube placement is recommended. Cortical mastoidectomy is performed in patients with recalcitrant infection or coalescent disease. Patients who are postmeningitis should be followed closely for hearing loss, as most develop a degree of labyrinthitis ossificans.[56]

*Lateral sinus thrombosis* presents with headache, high spiking fevers (often referred to as picket fence fevers), otalgia, and malodorous otorrhea.[57–60] Thrombophlebitis of the mastoid emissary vein results in edema and tenderness over the mastoid, described as the Griesinger sign. The development of diplopia, retro-orbital headaches, proptosis, and chemosis suggest cavernous sinus involvement. Diagnosis is made by MRI or CT, with an occluded sinus showing persistent dural enhancement with a central filling defect, termed the empty delta sign. Lumbar puncture should be performed unless contraindicated. Intracranial pressure should elevate with jugular vein occlusion but will not change when the ipsilateral jugular is compressed. Lateral sinus thrombosis is treated with intravenous antibiotics, with consideration for mastoidectomy with possible sinus decompression. The role of anticoagulation remains controversial.[61]

*Otitic hydrocephalus* consists of elevated intracranial pressure and otitis media. The condition presents similarly to idiopathic intracranial hypertension, with headache, nausea, and changes in vision. Treatment of the underlying otitis is essential for resolution. An *epidural abscess* may develop from direct extension of infection through a bony defect in the tegmen, which forms the boundary between the tympanic cavity and the middle fossa. Although often asymptomatic, epidural abscesses should be treated promptly with IV antibiotics and mastoidectomy to avoid spread to the brain parenchyma or subdural space.

An *otogenic brain abscess* classically presents with the triad of headache, fever, and focal neurologic deficit. Ataxia, nystagmus, or seizures may develop depending on the location of the abscess, and are often accompanied by headache and confusion secondary to increased intracranial pressure. Diagnosis is made by CT with contrast or MRI, demonstrating a ring-enhancing lesion with surrounding edema. With a high risk of lasting neurologic deficit, neurologic stabilization is the first priority in management. Broad-spectrum intravenous antibiotics, steroids, and myringotomy are initiated, with serial imaging to assess for response to treatment. Mastoidectomy is performed if there is remaining intratemporal infection. Management of the intracranial portion of the abscess is controversial and ranges from craniotomy and resection to aggressive medical management and aspiration.[54,62]

## SUMMARY

Chronic ear disease comprises a spectrum of otologic disorders, with presentations ranging from asymptomatic findings on physical examination to critically ill patients with intracranial complications. Although management of these conditions is typically surgical, primary care represents the first line in diagnosis, making awareness of these conditions essential and highlighting the importance of partnership between internists and otolaryngologists.

## REFERENCES

1. Buzi A, Gluth MB, Black B. Chronic ear disease in the modern era: evolution of treatment, epidemiology, and classification. In: Dornhoffer JL, Gluth MB, editors. The chronic ear. New York: Thieme; 2016. p. 2–7.
2. World Health Organization. Chronic suppurative otitis media: burden of illness and management options. Geneva (Switzerland): WHO; 2004.
3. Bluestone CD. Epidemiology and pathogenesis of chronic suppurative otitis media: implications for prevention and treatment. Int J Pediatr Otorhinolaryngol 1998;42(3):207–23.
4. Bluestone CD. Eustachian tube: structure, function, role in otitis media. Hamilton (Canada): PMPH-USA; 2005.

5. Sudhoff H. Eustachian tube dysfunction. 2nd edition. London: UNI-MED; 2017.
6. Vila PM, Thomas T, Liu C, et al. The burden and epidemiology of eustachian tube dysfunction in adults. Otolaryngol Head Neck Surg 2017;156(2):278–84.
7. Takahashi H, Honjo I, Fujita A. Endoscopic findings at the pharyngeal orifice of the eustachian tube in otitis media with effusion. Eur Arch Otorhinolaryngol 1996;253(1–2):42–4.
8. Poe DS, Gopen Q. Eustachian tube dysfunction. In: Snow JB, Wackym PA, Ballenger JJ, editors. Ballenger's otorhinolaryngology. New York: BC Decker; 2009. p. 201–8.
9. Sudhoff HH. Eustachian tube dysfunction, mucosal gas exchange, and effusion. In: Dornhoffer JL, Gluth MB, editors. The chronic ear. New York: Thieme; 2016. p. 8–13.
10. Lim DJ. Structure and function of the tympanic membrane: a review. Acta Otorhinolaryngol Belg 1995;49(2):101–15.
11. Podoshin L, Fradis M, Malatskey S, et al. Tympanoplasty in adults: a five-year survey. Ear Nose Throat J 1996;75(3):149–52, 155–6.
12. Poe DS. Diagnosis and management of the patulous eustachian tube. Otol Neurotol 2007;28(5):668–77.
13. Santa Maria PL. Tympanic membrane wound healing and epithelial migration. In: Dornhoffer JL, Gluth MB, editors. The chronic ear. New York: Thieme; 2016. p. 14–9.
14. Kristensen S. Spontaneous healing of traumatic tympanic membrane perforations in man: a century of experience. J Laryngol Otol 1992;106(12):1037–50.
15. Pau HW, Punke C, Just T. Tympanometric experiments on retracted ear drums— does tympanometry reflect the true middle ear pressure? Acta Otolaryngol 2009; 129(10):1080–7.
16. Sadé J, Berco E. Atelectasis and secretory otitis media. Ann Otol Rhinol Laryngol 1976;85(2 Suppl 25 Pt 2):66–72.
17. Tos M, Poulsen G. Attic retractions following secretory otitis. Acta Otolaryngol 1980;89(5–6):479–86.
18. Ohnishi T, Shirahata Y, Fukami M, et al. The atelectatic ear and its classification. Auris Nasus Larynx 1985;12(Suppl 1):S211–3.
19. Volkenstein S, Dazert S. Tubo-tympanic diseases: retraction, atelectasis, and middle ear effusion. In: Dornhoffer JL, Gluth MB, editors. The chronic ear. New York: Thieme; 2016. p. 111–7.
20. Podoshin L, Margalit A, Fradis M, et al. Cholesteatoma—an epidemiologic-study among members of Kibbutzim in Northern Israel. Ann Otol Rhinol Laryngol 1986; 95(4):365–8.
21. Benson J, Mwanri L. Chronic suppurative otitis media and cholesteatoma in Australia's refugee population. Aust Fam Physician 2012;41(12):978–80.
22. Michaels L. An epidermoid formation in the developing middle ear: possible source of cholesteatoma. J Otolaryngol 1986;15(3):169–74.
23. Persaud R, Hajioff D, Trinidade A, et al. Evidence-based review of aetiopathogenic theories of congenital and acquired cholesteatoma. J Laryngol Otol 2007;121(11):1013–9.
24. Hoppe F, Gluth MB. Pathophysiology of cholesteatoma. In: Dornhoffer JL, Gluth MB, editors. The chronic ear. New York: Thieme; 2016. p. 20–5.
25. House JW, Cunningham CD III. Otosclerosis. In: Flint PW, Haughey BH, Robbins KT, et al, editors. Cummings otolaryngology - head and neck surgery. 6th edition. Philadelphia: Elsevier Health Sciences; 2014. p. 2211–9.
26. Pichichero ME. Otitis media. Pediatr Clin North Am 2013;60(2):391–407.

27. Chonmaitree T. Viral and bacterial interaction in acute otitis media. Pediatr Infect Dis J 2000;19(5 Suppl):S24–30.
28. Ahn JH, Kim M-N, Suk YA, et al. Preoperative, intraoperative, and postoperative results of bacterial culture from patients with chronic suppurative otitis media. Otol Neurotol 2012;33(1):54–9.
29. Yeo SG, Park DC, Hong SM, et al. Bacteriology of chronic suppurative otitis media–a multicenter study. Acta Otolaryngol 2007;127(10):1062–7.
30. Brook I. The role of anaerobic bacteria in chronic suppurative otitis media in children: implications for medical therapy. Anaerobe 2008;14(6):297–300.
31. Park MK, Jung MH, Kang HJ, et al. The changes of MRSA infections in chronic suppurative otitis media. Otolaryngol Head Neck Surg 2008;139(3):395–8.
32. Adoga AA, Bakari A, Afolabi OA, et al. Bacterial isolates in chronic suppurative otitis media: a changing pattern? Niger J Med 2011;20(1):96–8.
33. Prakash R, Juyal D, Negi V, et al. Microbiology of chronic suppurative otitis media in a tertiary care setup of uttarakhand state, India. N Am J Med Sci 2013;5(4): 282–7.
34. Vaamonde P, Castro C, García-Soto N, et al. Tuberculous otitis media: a significant diagnostic challenge. Otolaryngol Head Neck Surg 2004;130(6):759–66.
35. Chole RA, Faddis BT. Evidence for microbial biofilms in cholesteatomas. Arch Otolaryngol Head Neck Surg 2002;128(10):1129–33.
36. Lee MR, Pawlowski KS, Luong A, et al. Biofilm presence in humans with chronic suppurative otitis media. Otolaryngol Head Neck Surg 2009;141(5):567–71.
37. Hoa M, Syamal M, Schaeffer MA, et al. Biofilms and chronic otitis media: an initial exploration into the role of biofilms in the pathogenesis of chronic otitis media. Am J Otolaryngol 2010;31(4):241–5.
38. Saunders J, Murray M, Alleman A. Biofilms in chronic suppurative otitis media and cholesteatoma: scanning electron microscopy findings. Am J Otolaryngol 2011;32(1):32–7.
39. Gu X, Keyoumu Y, Long L, et al. Detection of bacterial biofilms in different types of chronic otitis media. Eur Arch Otorhinolaryngol 2013;271(11):2877–83.
40. Post JC, Hiller NL, Nistico L, et al. The role of biofilms in otolaryngologic infections: update 2007. Curr Opin Otolaryngol Head Neck Surg 2007;15(5):347–51.
41. Wang EW, Agostini G, Olomu O, et al. Gentian violet and ferric ammonium citrate disrupt *Pseudomonas aeruginosa* biofilms. Laryngoscope 2008;118(11):2050–6.
42. Cho Y-S, Lee H-S, Kim S-W, et al. Tuberculous otitis media: a clinical and radiologic analysis of 52 patients. Laryngoscope 2006;116(6):921–7.
43. Penido Nde O, Chandrasekhar SS, Borin A, et al. Complications of otitis media - a potentially lethal problem still present. Braz J Otorhinolaryngol 2016;82(3): 253–62.
44. Levine SC, De Souza C, Shinners MJ. Intracranial complications of otitis media. In: Gulya AJ, Minor LB, Glasscock ME, et al, editors. Glasscock-Shambaugh surgery of the ear. 6th edition. Shelton, CT: People's Medical Publishing House; 2010. p. 451.
45. Dubey SP, Larawin V, Molumi CP. Intracranial spread of chronic middle ear suppuration. Am J Otolaryngol 2010;31(2):73–7.
46. Sanna M, Zini C, Bacciu S, et al. Management of the labyrinthine fistula in cholesteatoma surgery. ORL J Otorhinolaryngol Relat Spec 1984;46(3):165–72.
47. Geerse S, de Wolf MJF, Ebbens FA, et al. Management of labyrinthine fistula: hearing preservation versus prevention of residual disease. Eur Arch Otorhinolaryngol 2017;274(10):3605–12.

48. Carlson ML, Haynes DS, Wanna GB. Intratemporal and intracranial complications of otitis media. In: Dornhoffer JL, Gluth MB, editors. The chronic ear. New York: Thieme; 2016. p. 125–32.
49. Redaelli de Zinis LO, Gamba P, Balzanelli C. Acute otitis media and facial nerve paralysis in adults. Otol Neurotol 2003;24(1):113–7.
50. Carlson ML, Copeland WR, Driscoll CL, et al. Temporal bone encephalocele and cerebrospinal fluid fistula repair utilizing the middle cranial fossa or combined mastoid-middle cranial fossa approach. J Neurosurg 2013;119(5):1314–22.
51. Sanna M, Fois P, Paolo F, et al. Management of meningoencephalic herniation of the temporal bone: personal experience and literature review. Laryngoscope 2009;119(8):1579–85.
52. Dubey SP, Larawin V. Complications of chronic suppurative otitis media and their management. Laryngoscope 2007;117(2):264–7.
53. Migirov L, Duvdevani S, Kronenberg J. Otogenic intracranial complications: a review of 28 cases. Acta Otolaryngol 2005;125(8):819–22.
54. Wanna GB, Dharamsi LM, Moss JR, et al. Contemporary management of intracranial complications of otitis media. Otol Neurotol 2010;31(1):111–7.
55. Brouwer MC, McIntyre P, Prasad K, et al. Corticosteroids for acute bacterial meningitis. Cochrane Database Syst Rev 2015;(9):CD004405.
56. van Loon MC, Hensen EF, de Foer B, et al. Magnetic resonance imaging in the evaluation of patients with sensorineural hearing loss caused by meningitis: implications for cochlear implantation. Otol Neurotol 2013;34(5):845–54.
57. Novoa E, Podvinec M, Angst R, et al. Paediatric otogenic lateral sinus thrombosis: therapeutic management, outcome and thrombophilic evaluation. Int J Pediatr Otorhinolaryngol 2013;77(6):996–1001.
58. Seven H, Ozbal AE, Turgut S. Management of otogenic lateral sinus thrombosis. Am J Otolaryngol 2004;25(5):329–33.
59. Wong BYW, Hickman S, Richards M, et al. Management of paediatric otogenic cerebral venous sinus thrombosis: a systematic review. Clin Otolaryngol 2015; 40(6):704–14.
60. de Oliveira Penido N, Testa JRG, Inoue DP, et al. Presentation, treatment, and clinical course of otogenic lateral sinus thrombosis. Acta Otolaryngol 2009; 129(7):729–34.
61. Bradley DT, Hashisaki GT, Mason JC. Otogenic sigmoid sinus thrombosis: what is the role of anticoagulation? Laryngoscope 2002;112(10):1726–9.
62. Hafidh MA, Keogh I, Walsh RMC, et al. Otogenic intracranial complications. A 7-year retrospective review. Am J Otolaryngol 2006;27(6):390–5.

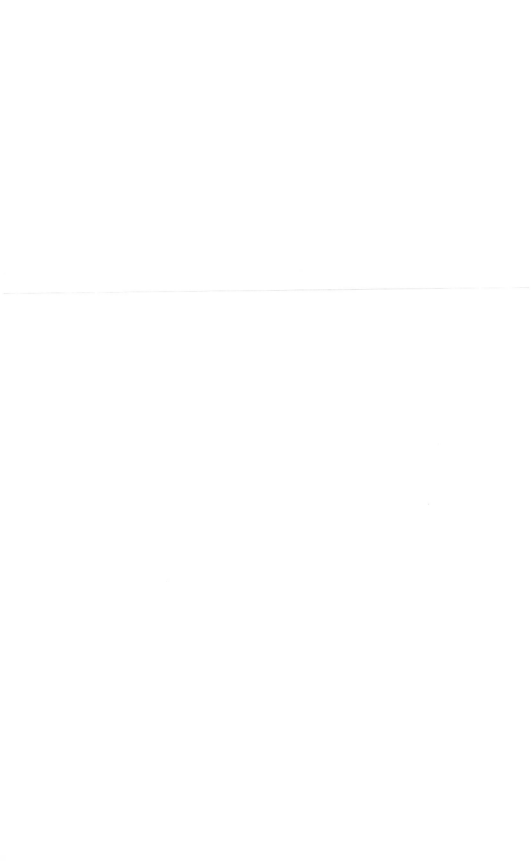

# Tinnitus

Divya A. Chari, MD, Charles J. Limb, MD*

## KEYWORDS

- Objective tinnitus • Subjective tinnitus • Audiogram
- Abnormal perception of sounds • Pulsatile tinnitus • Cognitive behavioral therapy
- Hearing aids

## KEY POINTS

- Tinnitus is divided into objective and subjective forms. The former refers to tinnitus that may be perceived by the examiner, whereas the latter is heard only by the patient.
- Subjective tinnitus is often associated with hearing loss.
- If the history, physical examination, and/or audiogram raise suspicion for an underlying disease process, directed imaging and additional testing should be performed.
- Treatment of tinnitus should be tailored based on the severity of the tinnitus experience.

## INTRODUCTION

Tinnitus is the perception of sound in the absence of an external acoustic stimulus. Tinnitus is a common and occasionally debilitating medical condition. With an estimated prevalence of 10% to 15% in adults, tinnitus is thought to affect more than 50 million people in the United States.[1] Approximately 25% of adults who experience tinnitus report that the condition interferes with daily activity and 1% to 3% of individuals report that their quality of life is severely affected.

The term tinnitus originates from the Latin word "tinnire," which means "to ring."[2] Although tinnitus often manifests as ringing, in fact the condition encompasses any phantom percept and may present as buzzing, roaring, whistling, hissing, or variable combinations of these descriptions. Tinnitus may be unilateral or bilateral, pulsatile or nonpulsatile, intermittent or constant. The perceived intensity may also vary. Although most patients with tinnitus are less severely affected, some experience anxiety, depression, and extreme life changes. Prompt identification and intervention is required in patients who have tinnitus accompanied by severe anxiety or depression because suicide has been reported in patients with tinnitus who have a comorbid psychiatric illness.[3]

Tinnitus has many possible causes; a thorough history and physical examination should be conducted to identify any underlying disorder. Frequently reported causes

Relevant Disclosures: None.

Department of Otolaryngology–Head and Neck Surgery, University of California San Francisco, 2233 Post Street, 3rd Floor, San Francisco, CA 94115, USA

* Corresponding author.

E-mail address: Charles.Limb@ucsf.edu

include sensorineural hearing loss (SNHL) attributable to aging, prolonged noise exposure, and head injury. Tinnitus has also been associated with otologic diseases including otosclerosis and endolymphatic hydrops (Meniere disease). Some studies have suggested a small genetic predisposition.[4] Various drugs have been shown to trigger tinnitus, including aminoglycoside antibiotics; salicylates; loop diuretics; quinine; and chemotherapeutics, such as methotrexate and cisplatin.[5] Rarely, tinnitus is a manifestation of a serious disease, such as vestibular schwannoma or vascular tumor. In general, pulsatile tinnitus, unilateral tinnitus, and tinnitus associated with other unilateral otologic symptoms (eg, hearing loss or vertigo) are more commonly associated with underlying disease processes in comparison with bilateral tinnitus.

Tinnitus is divided into two categories: objective and subjective. Subjective tinnitus, which comprises most cases, is the perception of sound in the absence of an identifiable acoustic source and is heard only by the patient. Objective tinnitus refers to the generation of noise (somatosounds) near the ear caused by vascular or neurologic disorders or eustachian tube dysfunction. In some cases of objective tinnitus, the examiner may actually hear the sounds, typically through turbulent blood flow or spontaneous contractions of the muscles in the soft palate or middle ear.

This article outlines current knowledge of tinnitus, describes the work-up and evaluation of tinnitus, reviews its commonly associated diseases, and discusses established and emerging treatment approaches.

## PATHOPHYSIOLOGY OF TINNITUS

The complex pathophysiologic mechanism by which tinnitus is produced remains poorly understood. Tinnitus may originate at any location along the auditory pathway from the external ear to the auditory cortex. One leading theory is that although cochlear abnormalities may be the initial source of tinnitus, a subsequent cascade of neural changes in the central auditory cortex perpetuates the symptoms of tinnitus.[6] This theory is supported by functional MRI studies indicating that a loss of cochlear input to neurons in the central auditory system can result in abnormal neural activity in the auditory cortex or inferior colliculus.[7,8] Levine[9] suggests that a reduction of auditory nerve input leads to disinhibition of the dorsal cochlear nucleus and a subsequent increase in spontaneous activity in the central auditory cortex, which is perceived as tinnitus. This idea is known as the dorsal cochlear nucleus hypothesis. Several studies have suggested that the reorganization of pathways in the central nervous system that occurs in tinnitus is similar to that observed in neuropathic pain.[8]

## DIAGNOSTIC EVALUATION OF TINNITUS
### History

Conceptually, it is helpful to characterize the tinnitus as objective or subjective, because this determination drives additional work-up and treatment. Based on the patient's description of the sounds, it is often possible to determine whether the tinnitus is a result of an identifiable somatosound. For example, pulsatile tinnitus that is synchronous with the heartbeat is suggestive of a vascular cause, whereas clicking or low-pitched buzzing may be indicative of palatal myoclonus or contractions of the tensor tympani or stapedius muscle. Tinnitus of vascular origin may be exacerbated by physical exercise and modulated by compression or rotation of the neck. By contrast, subjective tinnitus is less likely to be affected by changes in head position.

The examiner should question the patient to determine such characteristics as the duration of symptoms, laterality, exacerbating and alleviating factors, and persistence (constant vs intermittent). It is also important to determine how bothersome the tinnitus is to the patient, because treatment options differ depending on the perceived severity of the condition. Health questionnaires, such as the tinnitus handicap inventory and the tinnitus functional index, help assess the effects.

A complete otologic history includes questions regarding subjective hearing loss, vertigo, otalgia, otorrhea, aural fullness, autophony (increased resonance of one's own voice), childhood ear infections, noise exposure, prior otologic surgeries, and family history of hearing disorders. Because tinnitus is occasionally associated with medical conditions, other pertinent information includes a previous history of cancer or chemotherapy, strokes, vascular malformations, blood pressure, thyroid disorders, migraines, anxiety, and depression.

### Physical Examination

The evaluation of tinnitus requires a complete head and neck examination, including a careful otoscopic examination, assessment of cranial nerve function, tuning fork testing, and vestibular testing when appropriate. If the patient complains of a pulse-synchronous sound, auscultation should be performed over the mastoid process, preauricular region, and carotid arteries. Ipsilateral compression of the internal jugular vein may suppress tinnitus of venous origin. Otoscopic examination reveals abnormalities of the external ear, ear canal, and tympanic membrane and middle ear space, whereas the Weber and Rinne tests suggest either a sensorineural or conductive hearing loss.

### Audiogram

All patients with tinnitus should undergo audiometric assessment. Diagnostic testing should include the following components:

1. Measurement of pure tone thresholds
2. Speech audiometry
3. Tympanometry
4. Acoustic reflex testing

The conventional audiogram assesses the threshold at which the patient is able to detect pure tones varying in frequency from 250 to 8000 Hz. In adults, normal hearing is defined as a threshold of less than 20 dB at all frequencies tested. Speech audiometry determines the lowest intensity level at which speech stimuli (spondees) is repeated 50% of the time (speech recognition threshold) and the percentage of words that are repeated correctly when presented at a suprathreshold level (speech discrimination test). The acoustic reflex refers to an involuntary muscle contraction of the stapedius muscle in response to an ipsilateral or contralateral acoustic stimulus. An absent acoustic reflex is consistent with a middle ear conductive abnormality or a retrocochlear abnormality. However, in patients with air-bone gaps on pure tone testing and intact acoustic reflexes, a third mobile window syndrome, such as superior semicircular canal dehiscence, may be suspected.

Additional audiologic measurements of tinnitus include pitch masking, loudness matching, extended high-frequency audiometry, and minimum masking level. These measurements provide quantitative information about the characteristics of the tinnitus and may help predict whether the patient's tinnitus will be successfully masked by an external noise.

### Imaging and Additional Testing

The work-up of tinnitus involves a complete history; physical examination; audiogram; and, if an underlying disease is suspected, additional diagnostic testing or imaging (**Table 1**). Laboratory tests should be ordered depending on diseases suspected

**Table 1**
**Ancillary diagnostic testing in evaluation of tinnitus**

|  | Type of Tinnitus | Ancillary Diagnostic Testing |
|---|---|---|
| Objective | Vascular cause | Contrast-enhanced CT scan of temporal bones |
|  |  | Carotid duplex ultrasound and/or MR angiography |
|  | Patulous eustachian tube | Flexible endoscopic examination of nasopharynx |
|  | Palatal myoclonus | Contrast-enhanced MRI scan of brain |
|  | Stapedial or tensor tympani myoclonus | Contrast-enhanced MRI scan of brain |
| Subjective | Symmetric, bilateral tinnitus with associated sensorineural hearing loss | No further evaluation required |
|  | Unilateral or asymmetric tinnitus or hearing loss | Contrast-enhanced MRI of brain and IAC to evaluate for retrocochlear lesion |
|  | Tinnitus associated with conductive hearing loss | CT scan of temporal bones if suspected ossicular abnormality |
|  | Tinnitus caused by Meniere disease | Contrast-enhanced MRI may be required to rule out retrocochlear lesion |
|  | Tinnitus caused by superior semicircular canal dehiscence | CT scan of temporal bones. VEMP testing |

*Abbreviations:* CT, computed tomography; IAC, internal auditory canal; VEMP, vestibular evoked myogenic potential.

based on the preliminary history and head and neck examination. Such laboratory tests may include thyroid function tests, complete blood count, and lipid profile, among others.

Typically, imaging is not necessary in the work-up of subjective tinnitus that is non-lateralizing and associated with symmetric hearing loss. Imaging should be performed, however, when a pulsatile or retrocochlear lesion is suspected or in cases of cranial nerve dysfunction, that is, facial paralysis or paralysis of the glossopharyngeal, vagus, and spinal accessory cranial nerves (Vernet syndrome). Imaging of choice for a pulsatile lesion is either computed tomography (CT) angiography or magnetic resonance angiography. Unilateral tinnitus associated with asymmetric hearing loss suggests the possibility of a retrocochlear lesion, such as a vestibular schwannoma or meningioma, and MRI of the brain and internal auditory canals with and without gadolinium is necessary to confirm or rule out these diagnoses. Patients with these findings may undergo additional tests to locate and characterize the lesion, including auditory brainstem evoked responses, tone decay, reflex decay, and measures of vestibular function.

## CLASSIFICATION OF TINNITUS
### Objective Tinnitus

The first step in the evaluation of objective tinnitus is to determine whether the somatosound is caused by an abnormally heightened perception of a normal somatosound or an abnormally produced somatosound (**Table 2**).

### Vascular cause

Vascular disorders associated with tinnitus may be subdivided into arterial and venous types. Arterial abnormalities may be associated with pulse-synchronous somatosounds. Physical examination may reveal an audible bruit in the neck or near the ear. If a carotid bruit is suspected, a carotid ultrasound followed by a CT scan with

**Table 2**
**Classification of tinnitus and selected examples**

| Type of Tinnitus | Examples |
|---|---|
| Objective | Conductive hearing loss (cerumen impaction, ossicular discontinuity, cholesteatoma)<br>Third window anomalies (SSCD)<br>Vascular anomalies<br>Patulous eustachian tube<br>Palatal myoclonus<br>Stapedial or tensor tympani myoclonus |
| Subjective | Idiopathic, often secondary to sensorineural hearing loss<br>Conductive hearing loss<br>Endolymphatic hydrops (Meniere disease)<br>Third window anomalies (SSCD)<br>Tumors (vestibular schwannomas, meningiomas)<br>Somatic tinnitus (related to temporomandibular joint dysfunction or cervical dysfunction) |

intravenous contrast or MRI with gadolinium is recommended. Treatment options include arterial ligation, embolization, and decompression via middle fossa or posterior fossa (suboccipital) approach.[10]

Venous abnormalities associated with tinnitus include sigmoid sinus wall anomalies, transverse sinus stenosis, idiopathic intracranial hypertension, and a high or dehiscent jugular bulb. A CT scan with delayed contrast injection for venous enhancement can reveal these conditions.[11] Tinnitus associated with venous abnormalities may present as a soft, low-pitched hum and decrease with compression of the ipsilateral jugular vein.

Tumors of the middle ear and jugular foramen may be identified by otoscopic examination or the presence of lower cranial nerve dysfunction. A middle ear paraganglioma (glomus tympanicum) does not necessitate further imaging if it is visualized circumferentially on otoscopy. Patients with glomus jugulare tumors may present with voice and swallowing problems caused by deficits in the lower cranial nerves. Treatment of these tumors involves a combination of angiography for preoperative embolization and surgical resection via lateral skull base approach. Arteriovenous malformations and fistulae can also cause pulsatile tinnitus. Treatment of these conditions is important because they carry a risk of intracerebral hemorrhage.[12] The role of vascular loop compression of the eighth cranial nerve has been debated in the literature, but one systematic review showed that such loops are 80 times more common in patients with pulsatile tinnitus than those with nonpulsatile tinnitus.[13]

### Palatal myoclonus

Palatal myoclonus is characterized by involuntary contractions of the soft palate, causing bilateral clicking tinnitus. The myoclonus is rapid and irregular with a rate between 40 and 200 beats per minute. The examiner may be able to hear the sound described by the patient when listening near the patient's external auditory canal or with a stethoscope at the lateral neck. Inspection of the palate reveals myoclonic jerks and a nasal endoscopy may be necessary. Occipital headaches or temporomandibular joint pain are common comorbid conditions. Two types of palatal myoclonus have been described. In symptomatic palatal myoclonus, the disease process is the result of a brainstem lesion, typically involving the upper cerebellar peduncle (the dentate-rubro-olivary triangle of Guillain-Mollaret).[14] When no discrete lesion is identified, the condition is termed essential palatal myoclonus. Patients presenting with new-onset palatal myoclonus should be evaluated with an MRI of the brain and brainstem to assess for a localized lesion. Treatment options include antispasmodic agents and muscle relaxants, such as clonazepam or diazepam, and antiseizure medications, such as lamotrigine, valproate, and carbamazepine. Additionally, botulinum toxin injections have been shown to provide temporary relief.[15]

### Stapedial or tensor tympani myoclonus

Middle ear myoclonus may cause tinnitus from abnormal contraction of the tensor tympani or stapedius muscles in the absence of acoustic stimuli. Idiopathic stapedial muscle contractions may cause a fluttering or buzzing sound to be heard on facial movement.[16] This pathology is sometimes seen in patients recovering from Bell palsy. When the affected side of the face contracts, the ipsilateral stapedius muscle contracts concurrently, likely through synkinesis caused by aberrant facial nerve regeneration.[17]

Irregular, intermittent, unilateral tinnitus, termed "typewriter" tinnitus, may be a sign of aberrant contraction of the tensor tympani muscle. This type of tinnitus has been found to respond to carbamazepine.[18]

### Patulous eustachian tube dysfunction

Patulous eustachian tube dysfunction is a condition where the eustachian tube remains pathologically patent. Patients with this disease process often report autophony, aural fullness, and a wave-like tinnitus that is synchronous with respiration. Diagnosis is made with otoscopic examination, which reveals a tympanic membrane that moves synchronously with respiration.[19] This condition has been shown to develop following significant weight loss, possibly because of loss of peritubal fat tissue.[20] It has also been associated with pregnancy and a history of radiation therapy to or near the nasopharynx.

Although no standard of treatment has been established for patulous eustachian tube, several measures have been moderately successful in alleviating symptoms. Estrogen nasal drops, oral administration of saturated solution of potassium iodide has been used to induce swelling of the eustachian tube opening. Topical nasal medication containing diluted hydrochloric acid, chlorobutanol, and benzyl alcohol is effective in some patients.[21] Myringotomy and tympanostomy tube insertions reduce symptoms temporarily, but do not provide definitive treatment.[22] Another strategy is to inject Vox implants, cartilage, or autologous fat tissue into the torus tubarius.[20,23]

### Subjective Tinnitus

Primary idiopathic tinnitus is a diagnosis of exclusion (**Fig. 1**). Primary tinnitus describes tinnitus that is idiopathic with or without concurrent SNHL, whereas secondary tinnitus refers to tinnitus associated with an identifiable organic condition. The organic condition in question could be simple cerumen impaction of the external auditory canal, eustachian tube dysfunction, middle ear pathology, Meniere disease, superior semicircular canal dehiscence, or vestibular schwannomas (see **Table 2**).

A comprehensive history, physical examination, and audiogram must confirm the absence of other disease processes. For example, if tinnitus lateralizes to one ear, is associated with asymmetric hearing loss or other focal neurologic abnormalities, or has an abrupt onset in association with sudden hearing loss or vertigo, diagnostic imaging should be obtained to exclude a retrocochlear lesion.[24] In cases where subjective tinnitus arises from conductive hearing loss (ie, ossicular chain dislocation, otosclerosis, cholesteatoma), the history, physical examination, and audiogram are often indicative of the underlying condition. Although imaging is not strictly necessary,

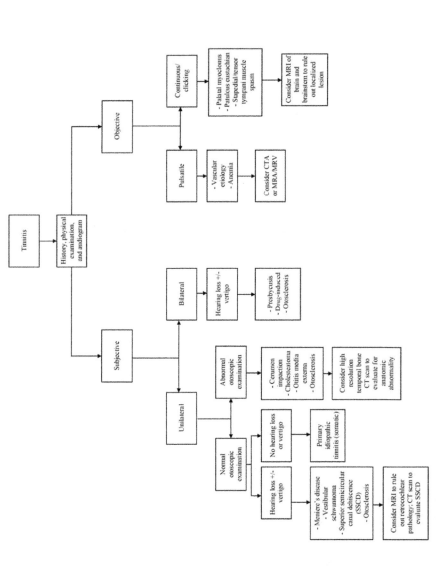

**Fig. 1.** Suggested diagnostic algorithm for work-up of tinnitus. CTA, computed tomography angiogram; MRA, magnetic resonance angiogram; MRV, magentic resonance venogram. (*Adapted from* Crummer RW, Hassan GA. Diagnostic approach to tinnitus. Am Fam Physician 2004;69(1):24; with permission.)

the surgeon may prefer to obtain a high-resolution CT scan of the temporal bone before intervention to evaluate for any anatomic abnormalities.

Psychiatric illness and sleep disturbance are often associated with severe tinnitus. The initial history and physical examination should include evaluation of possible associated depression and anxiety. If identified, the examiner should consider referring the patient to mental health professionals for assessment and treatment.

## TREATMENT OF TINNITUS

Despite its widespread prevalence, tinnitus largely remains a clinical enigma. When tinnitus is a symptom of a distinct disease process, treatment of that process resolves the condition; otherwise, treatment must be tailored based on the severity of the tinnitus experience. For patients with mild tinnitus, it may suffice to provide the diagnosis and explain the natural history and progression of the condition.

The following review of treatment options is primarily for patients with bothersome, persistent ($\geq$6 months) tinnitus. No single cure for tinnitus exists, which is at least partly because of the multidimensional clinical characteristics of tinnitus and the low consistency in outcome measurement. In general, current treatment strategies for tinnitus have been aimed at improving quality of life for patients.

### Psychological Treatments

#### Counseling and psychoeducation
Although many cases of tinnitus cannot be cured, counseling and psychoeducation help patients cope with tinnitus and its potential consequences, such as emotional distress, sleep disturbance, and disruption to their occupation and personal lives.

#### Tinnitus retraining therapy
The goal of tinnitus retraining therapy is to "retrain" the brain to habituate to the tinnitus signal and thereby encourage the patient perceive the tinnitus as a neutral stimulus.[25] Tinnitus retraining therapy involves two major components: directive, or educational, counseling; and sound therapy in the form of masking, or white noise, devices set slightly below the level of the patient's perceived tinnitus. Although some studies have suggested beneficial effects,[26,27] a Cochrane meta-analysis was unable to draw firm conclusions because of the absence of high-quality randomized clinical trials.[28]

#### Cognitive behavioral therapy
Cognitive behavioral therapy (CBT) attempts to reduce the undesirable emotional and behavioral responses to tinnitus by restructuring the patient's maladaptive thoughts and behaviors. The main components of CBT are psychoeducation, relaxation training, mindfulness-based training, imagery training, and exposure therapy. Several systematic reviews have suggested that CBT helps mitigate the condition.[29–31] In particular, one meta-analysis found that CBT offers a significant reduction of depression and increase in quality of life in eight trials (468 patients), but did not find any effect on subjective tinnitus loudness in six trials.[32]

### Auditory Stimulation

#### Sound therapy
Masking devices produce white noise that is intended to be relaxing and reduce the perception of tinnitus. Masking attempts to alleviate the perceived loudness of tinnitus by decreasing tinnitus-related hypersynchronous activity within the auditory cortex through the attraction of lateral inhibition. In particular, notched sound therapy is a

tailored form of sound therapy where the frequency of tinnitus is removed from the sound stimulus.[33–35] Since the introduction of sound therapy in the 1970s,[36] two general types of sound therapy approaches have emerged: total masking and partial masking. Because prolonged exposure to broadband (total) masking stimulation is thought to increase the risk for hearing loss, devices with adjustable, frequency-specific narrowband (partial) masking have become popular.[37] Custom sound generators that may be worn behind the ear, similarly to a hearing aid, are available. Additionally, some hearing aids have integrated sound generators, which is ideal for patients who suffer from hearing loss in addition to tinnitus.[31]

### Hearing aids
Hearing aids are often helpful in the treatment of tinnitus, particularly given the high incidence of concurrent hearing loss in patient with tinnitus. Hearing aids amplify ambient environmental noise, which can have the effect of masking tinnitus. Although hearing aids are widely used, the beneficial effect of hearing aids is more pronounced in patients with a tinnitus at a frequency less than 6000 Hz (ie, within the amplification range of hearing aids).[38,39] Hearing aids with built-in sound generator devices can generate narrowband or broadband noise and provide adequate masking in the high-frequency region.

### Cochlear implants
In general, surgical intervention has not been found to be successful in tinnitus treatment apart from addressing specific underlying conditions, such as otosclerosis or vestibular schwannomas. Cochlear implantation, however, is a viable treatment option for patients with bilateral profound SNHL and concurrent tinnitus, with reports that tinnitus is eliminated in more than 80% of cases.[39–41] Patients responded equally well regardless of the type of tinnitus.

Additionally, preliminary studies suggest that cochlear implantation successfully suppresses tinnitus in patients with single-sided profound SNHL and normal or near-normal hearing in the contralateral ear. Preliminary studies suggest that tinnitus suppression is successful in this subgroup.[42,43] As unilateral cochlear implantation for single sided hearing loss with tinnitus becomes more common, this may also be an effective option for severe unilateral tinnitus.

## Pharmacologic Treatments

Many medications have been used to treat tinnitus medically, but currently no drug is approved by the Food and Drug Administration for the treatment of primary, idiopathic tinnitus. Most of the drugs tested are ineffective, and many have unwanted side effects.

### Antidepressants
Tricyclic antidepressants and selective serotonin reuptake inhibitors have been studied for the treatment of tinnitus. Several trials have shown improvement of tinnitus measures with antidepressants, but given the methodologic limitations of these studies and lack of generalizability to patients without depression, antidepressants are not typically recommended for the treatment of tinnitus.[24] Amitriptyline has been found to significantly reduce tinnitus complaints and tinnitus loudness compared with placebo.[44] Another study investigating the effect of nortriptyline on patients with severe tinnitus and major depression found that depression and tinnitus loudness levels were decreased.[45] One study noted improvement in tinnitus loudness and severity with sertraline in patients with comorbid depression and anxiety.[46] However, paroxetine was found to have no effect on the improvement of tinnitus symptoms in patients with chronic tinnitus without comorbid depression.[47] Taken collectively, these

data suggest that patients with tinnitus with depression and anxiety may benefit from antidepressants, but that antidepressants should not routinely be used as treatment of chronic tinnitus.

### Anxiolytics
Clinical trials investigating the effect of anxiolytics, such as benzodiazepines, on tinnitus do not consistently show benefit. In one double-blind placebo-controlled study, alprazolam reduced tinnitus loudness, but the study suffered from a small sample size of the study and lack of replication. Additionally, these medications can have adverse effects, including a high risk of drug dependency and drowsiness.

### Anticonvulsants
Anticonvulsant drugs, such as lamotrigine and carbamazepine, potentially suppress central auditory hyperactivity related to tinnitus. However, a Cochrane review failed to demonstrate preponderance of benefit over harm. Side effects of anticonvulsants include nauseas, dizziness, and headaches.

### Other compounds
Ginkgo biloba contains bioactive flavonoids with vasoactive and antioxidant properties and is the most commonly used herbal supplement for tinnitus. Even though some studies have suggested beneficial effects of gingko on tinnitus, particularly in patients with short-duration symptoms, there is growing evidence from randomized controlled trials that gingko is no more effective in alleviating tinnitus symptoms than placebo.[48] Several other dietary supplements have been studied, such as B-complex vitamins[49] and melatonin,[50] but no beneficial effects have been noted.

### Brain Stimulation
Transcranial magnetic stimulation is a technique in which brief magnetic pulses are delivered via a coil to specific areas of the brain through an intact scalp. Repetitive transcranial magnetic stimulation (rTMS) has been shown to reduce neuronal activity in directly stimulated areas of the brain and structurally connected remote areas. Because tinnitus perception has been associated with abnormal activity in the central auditory system, rTMS was proposed as a way to treat tinnitus. Although some studies have shown improvements in tinnitus severity with rTMS,[51,52] randomized controlled trials and systematic reviews have not demonstrated a long-term benefit in the reduction of tinnitus or improvements in patient quality of life.[53,54]

Epidural stimulation of the secondary auditory cortex by implanted electrodes produces tinnitus suppression in some patients[55] and emerging data suggest that deep brain stimulation of the caudate nucleus may have a beneficial effect in the treatment of tinnitus.[56]

## SUMMARY AND FUTURE CONSIDERATIONS

Tinnitus is a complex and heterogenous disorder affecting at least 1 in 10 people. A thorough history, complete physical examination, and audiogram are essential for all patients suffering from tinnitus. If specific findings are noted, further evaluation with imaging may be warranted. Often, a multidisciplinary approach is needed for comprehensive diagnostic assessment and therapeutic management. Referral to an otolaryngologist and audiologist can facilitate evaluation, treatment, and counseling. As yet, there are no proven cures for tinnitus, and management remains challenging. However, advances have been made in understanding the pathophysiology of the disease process, and exciting new research has identified potential therapeutic targets that could provide a path to reliable and long-term tinnitus suppression.

## REFERENCES

1. Henry JA, Dennis KC, Schechter MA. General review of tinnitus: prevalence, mechanisms, effects, and management. J Speech Lang Hear Res 2005;48(5): 1204–35.
2. Crummer RW, Hassan GA. Diagnostic approach to tinnitus. Am Fam Physician 2004;69(1):120–6.
3. Lewis J, Stephens S, McKenna L. Tinnitus and suicide. Clin Otolaryngol Allied Sci 1994;19(19):50–4.
4. Kvestad E, Czajkowski N, Engdahl B, et al. Low heritability of tinnitus: results from the second Nord-Trondelag health study. Arch Otolaryngol Head Neck Surg 2010;136(2):178–82.
5. Cianfrone G, Pentangelo D, Cianfrone F, et al. Pharmacological drugs inducing ototoxicity, vestibular symptoms and tinnitus: a reasoned and updated guide. Eur Rev Med Pharmacol Sci 2011;15(6):601–36.
6. Eggermont JJ, Roberts LE. The Neuroscience of Tinnitus: Understanding Abnormal and Normal Auditory Perception. Front Syst Neurosci 2012;6:53.
7. Melcher JR, Sigalovsky IS, Guinan JJ, et al. Lateralized tinnitus studied with functional magnetic resonance imaging: abnormal inferior colliculus activation. J Neurophysiol 2000;83(2):1058–72.
8. Lockwood AH, Salvi RJ, Coad ML, et al. The functional neuroanatomy of tinnitus: evidence for limbic system links and neural plasticity. Neurology 1998;50(1): 114–20.
9. Levine RA. Somatic (craniocervical) tinnitus and the dorsal cochlear nucleus hypothesis. Am J Otolaryngol 1999;20(6):351–62.
10. Herzog JA, Bailey S, Meyer J. Vascular loops of the internal auditory canal: a diagnostic dilemma. Am J Otol 1997;18(1):26–31.
11. Dong C, Zhao PF, Yang JG, et al. Incidence of vascular anomalies and variants associated with unilateral venous pulsatile tinnitus in 242 patients based on dual-phase contrast-enhanced computed tomography. Chin Med J (Engl) 2015;128(5):581–5.
12. King WA, Martin NA. Intracerebral hemorrhage due to dural arteriovenous malformations and fistulae. Neurosurg Clin N Am 1992;3(3):577–90.
13. Chadha NK, Weiner GM. Vascular loops causing otological symptoms: a systematic review and meta-analysis. Clin Otolaryngol 2008;33(1):5–11.
14. Pearce JMS. Palatal myoclonus (syn. palatal tremor). Eur Neurol 2008;60(6): 312–5.
15. Penney SE, Bruce IA, Saeed SR. Botulinum toxin is effective and safe for palatal tremor: a report of five cases and a review of the literature. J Neurol 2006;253(7): 857–60.
16. Marchiando A, Per-Lee JH, Jackson RT. Tinnitus due to idiopathic stapedial muscle spasm. Ear Nose Throat J 1983;62(1):8–13.
17. Levine RA, Oron Y. Tinnitus. Handb Clin Neurol 2015;129:409–31.
18. Levine RA. Typewriter tinnitus: a carbamazepine-responsive syndrome related to auditory nerve vascular compression. ORL J Otorhinolaryngol Relat Spec 2006; 68(1):43–6.
19. Hussein AA, Adams AS, Turner JH. Surgical management of patulous eustachian tube: a systematic review. Laryngoscope 2015;125(9):2193–8.

20. Poe DS. Diagnosis and management of the patulous eustachian tube. Otol Neurotol 2007;28(5):668–77.
21. Sudhoff HH, Mueller S. Treatment of pharyngotympanic tube dysfunction. Auris Nasus Larynx 2018;45(2):207–14.
22. Henry DF, DiBartolomeo JR. Patulous eustachian tube identification using tympanometry. J Am Acad Audiol 1993;4(1):53–7.
23. Schroder S, Lehmann M, Sudhoff H, et al. The patulous eustachian tube-novel surgical approaches. HNO 2013;61(12):1017–25 [in German].
24. Tunkel DE, Bauer CA, Sun GH, et al. Clinical practice guideline: tinnitus. Otolaryngol Head Neck Surg 2014;151(4):S1–40.
25. Jastreboff PJ, Hazell JW. A neurophysiological approach to tinnitus: clinical implications. Br J Audiol 1993;27:7–17.
26. Henry JA, Schechter MA, Zaugg TL, et al. Outcomes of clinical trial: tinnitus masking versus tinnitus retraining therapy. J Am Acad Audiol 2006;17(2):104–32.
27. Bauer CA, Brozoski TJ. Effect of tinnitus retraining therapy on the loudness and annoyance of tinnitus: a controlled trial. Ear Hear 2011;32(2):145–55.
28. Phillips J, Mcferran D. Tinnitus retraining therapy (TRT) for tinnitus. Cochrane Database Syst Rev 2010;3:CD007330.
29. Hesser H, Weise C, Westin VZ, et al. A systematic review and meta-analysis of randomized controlled trials of cognitive-behavioral therapy for tinnitus distress. Clin Psychol Rev 2010;31(4):545–53.
30. Andersson G, Lyttkens L. A meta-analytic review of psychological treatments for tinnitus. Br J Audiol 1999;33(4):201–10. Available at: http://www.embase.com/search/results?subaction=viewrecord&from=export&id=L29438479%5Cnhttp://sfx.library.uu.nl/utrecht?sid=EMBASE&issn=03005364&id=doi:&atitle=A+meta-analytic+review+of+psychological+treatments+for+tinnitus&stitle=Br.+J.+Audiol.&title=Brit.
31. Hoare DJ, Kowalkowski VL, Kang S, et al. Systematic review and meta-analyses of randomized controlled trials examining tinnitus management. Laryngoscope 2011;121(7):1555–64.
32. Martinez-Devesa P, Perera R, Theodoulou M, et al. Cognitive behavioural therapy for tinnitus. Cochrane Database Syst Rev 2010. https://doi.org/10.1002/14651858.CD005233.pub3.
33. Stracke H, Okamoto H, Pantev C. Customized notched music training reduces tinnitus loudness. Commun Integr Biol 2010;3(3):274–7.
34. Vernon J. Attemps to relieve tinnitus. J Am Audiol Soc 1977;2(4):124–31.
35. Vernon J, Schleuning A. Tinnitus: a new management. Laryngoscope 1978;88(3):413–9.
36. Schaette R, König O, Hornig D, et al. Acoustic stimulation treatments against tinnitus could be most effective when tinnitus pitch is within the stimulated frequency range. Hear Res 2010;269(1–2):95–101.
37. Hobson J, Chisholm EJ, Loveland ME. Sound therapy (masking) in the management of tinnitus in adults. Cochrane Database Syst Rev 2007;(1). https://doi.org/10.1002/14651858.CD006371.
38. McNeill C, Távora-Vieira D, Alnafjan F, et al. Tinnitus pitch, masking, and the effectiveness of hearing aids for tinnitus therapy. Int J Audiol 2012;51(12):914–9.
39. Bovo R, Ciorba A, Martini A. Tinnitus and cochlear implants. Auris Nasus Larynx 2011;38(1):14–20.
40. Baguley DM. New insights into tinnitus in cochlear implant recipients. Cochlear Implants Int 2010;11(Suppl. 2):31–6.

41. Kompis M, Pelizzone M, Dillier N, et al. Tinnitus before and 6 months after cochlear implantation. Audiol Neurootol 2012;17(3):161–8.
42. Punte AK, Meeus O, Van De Heyning P. Cochlear implants and tinnitus. In: Moller AR, langguth B, DeRidder D, et al, editors. Textbook of tinnitus. New York: Springer; 2011. p. 619–24.
43. Van De Heyning P, Vermeire K, Diebl M, et al. Incapacitating unilateral tinnitus in single-sided deafness treated by cochlear implantation. Ann Otol Rhinol Laryngol 2008;117(9):645–52.
44. Podoshin L, Ben-David Y, Fradis M, et al. Idiopathic subjective tinnitus treated by amitriptyline hydrochloride/biofeedback. Int Tinnitus J 1995;1(1):54–60.
45. Sullivan M, Katon W, Russo J, et al. A randomized trial of nortriptyline for severe chronic tinnitus: effects on depression, disability, and tinnitus symptoms. Arch Intern Med 1993;153(19):2251–9.
46. Kajsa-Mia H, Zöger S, Svedlund J, et al. The impact of sertraline on health-related quality of life in severe refractory tinnitus: a double-blind, randomized, placebo-controlled study. Audiol Med 2011;9(2):67–72.
47. Robinson SK, Viirre ES, Bailey KA, et al. Randomized placebo-controlled trial of a selective serotonin reuptake inhibitor in the treatment of nondepressed tinnitus subjects. Psychosom Med 2005;67(6):981–8.
48. Hilton MP, Zimmermann EF, Hunt WT. Ginkgo biloba for tinnitus. Cochrane Database Syst Rev 2013;(3):CD003852.
49. Shulman A. Subjective idiopathic tinnitus: a unified plan of management. Am J Otolaryngol 1992;13(2):63–74.
50. Rosenberg SI, Silverstein H, Rowan PT, et al. Effect of melatonin on tinnitus. Laryngoscope 1998;108(3):305–10.
51. Kleinjung T, Eichhammer P, Langguth B, et al. Long-term effects of repetitive transcranial magnetic stimulation (rTMS) in patients with chronic tinnitus. Otolaryngol Head Neck Surg 2005;132(4):566–9.
52. Rossi S, De Capua A, Ulivelli M, et al. Effects of repetitive transcranial magnetic stimulation on chronic tinnitus: a randomised, crossover, double blind, placebo controlled study. J Neurol Neurosurg Psychiatry 2007;78(8):857–63.
53. Piccirillo JF, Garcia KS, Nicklaus J, et al. Low-frequency repetitive transcranial magnetic stimulation to the temporoparietal junction for tinnitus. Arch Otolaryngol Head Neck Surg 2011;137(3):221.
54. Meng Z, Liu S, Zheng Y, et al. Repetitive transcranial magnetic stimulation for tinnitus. Cochrane Database Syst Rev 2011;(10):CD007946.
55. De Ridder D, Vanneste S, Kovacs S, et al. Transcranial magnetic stimulation and extradural electrodes implanted on secondary auditory cortex for tinnitus suppression. J Neurosurg 2011;114(4):903–11.
56. Cheung SW, Larson PS. Tinnitus modulation by deep brain stimulation in locus of caudate neurons (area LC). Neuroscience 2010;169(4):1768–78.

# Head and Neck Manifestations of Systemic Disease

Annie E. Moroco, BS, Johnathan D. McGinn, MD*

## KEYWORDS

- Otolaryngology • Systemic disease • Head and neck • Vasculitis • Laryngitis
- Sinusitis • Rheumatologic disease

## KEY POINTS

- Manifestations of systemic disease are common within the head and neck.
- Emergent complications of systemic disease may present in the head and neck and require timely referral to the otolaryngologist.
- Otolaryngologists can provide targeted therapy to improve head and neck symptoms of systemic disease.
- Systemic disease should be considered in the differential diagnosis for complaints of the head and neck.

## INTRODUCTION

Systemic diseases can affect the head and neck regions in a variety of focal and diffuse manners. These manifestations may be the initial indications of the systemic disease, or sequela of the established diagnosis. The symptoms and findings may share features of a variety of other systemic and local illnesses, thus making this distinction an important part of the evaluative process. An awareness of the possible head and neck presentations of underlying systemic disease is important in proper diagnosis but also key in those cases wherein complications or emergencies generated by the illness might be avoided or managed. This article describes several systemic diseases with various manifestations in the head and neck, highlighting those whose early presentations may help establish a diagnosis, or in which emergent complications may arise.

Disclosure Statement: No disclosures.
Division of Otolaryngology–Head and Neck Surgery, Department of Surgery, Penn State Milton S. Hershey Medical Center, 500 University Drive, Hershey, PA 17033, USA
* Corresponding author. Division of Otolaryngology–Head and Neck Surgery, 500 University Drive, PO Box 850, H091, Hershey, PA 17033.
E-mail address: jmcginn@pennstatehealth.psu.edu

Med Clin N Am 102 (2018) 1095–1107
https://doi.org/10.1016/j.mcna.2018.06.009
0025-7125/18/© 2018 Elsevier Inc. All rights reserved.

medical.theclinics.com

## Rheumatologic Disease

### Granulomatosis with polyangiitis

Granulomatosis with polyangiitis (GPA), formerly known as Wegener granulomatosis, is characterized by small vessel vasculitis and necrotizing granulomas of the upper airway, lung, and kidney. Compared with other vasculitides, GPA commonly manifests in the head and neck, and early presentation can mimic respiratory tract infection producing nasal and paranasal sinus symptoms of rhinosinusitis, rhinorrhea, crusting, and anosmia. Vasculitis can cause progressive damage to the sinonasal lining as well as underlying bone and cartilage. Typically, this manifests as nasal dryness, crusting, and even ulceration. This process may progress, resulting in perforation of the septum, and with loss of nasal support, a saddle nose deformity may occur. Manifestations of GPA in the ear include otitis media, otorrhea, polychondritis, and even sensorineural or conductive hearing loss. Although uncommon, strawberry gingivitis and poorly healing ulcerations of the oral cavity can present in patients with GPA. Damage to the maxilla and mandible can result in tooth mobility and loss of dentition. Laryngeal involvement with symptoms of hoarseness, cough, hemoptysis, and dyspnea is present in 10% to 20% of patients with GPA. Laryngeal GPA has predominant inflammation and scarring of the subglottic region causing narrowing of the airway. Subglottic stenosis presents with a stridor that is often mistaken for asthmatic wheeze.

The presence of serum cytoplasmic antineutrophilic cytoplasmic antibody or granuloma on biopsy confirms a diagnosis of GPA. Treatment of patients with GPA includes systemic corticosteroids and other immunosuppressant agents. Of concern from an otolaryngologic perspective is proper airway management. Progression of subglottic stenosis may require urgent surgical intervention, including intralesional steroid injection, dilation, or even tracheostomy. Sinonasal manifestations may be managed with local topical steroids sprays, nasal saline lavage, and in select cases, nasoseptal reconstruction or endoscopic sinus surgery.[1]

### Eosinophilic granulomatosis with polyangiitis

Eosinophilic granulomatosis with polyangiitis (EGPA), also known as Churg-Strauss syndrome, is a vasculitis affecting small and medium vessels characterized by a triphasic progression: (1) a prodromal stage of airway inflammation with allergic rhinitis and asthma, (2) an eosinophilic phase damaging the lungs or digestive tract, and (3) a life-threatening vasculitis phase causing systemic granulomatous inflammation. Like GPA, EGPA is characterized by chronic rhinosinusitis, but EGPA is distinct in its early presentation of nasal polyposis and asthma, less commonly progressing to septal perforation. In addition to nasal manifestations, EGPA may present with serous otitis media, sensorineural hearing loss, or destructive oral lesions. The presence of antineutrophilic cytoplasmic antibody is less common in EGPA than in other vasculitides, and the definitive diagnosis is based on necrotizing vasculitis with prominent eosinophilia seen on biopsy. Peripheral eosinophilia commonly characterizes the later stages of the disease. Glucocorticoids are the standard treatment of EGPA with other immunosuppressants and biologics being options.[2]

### Sarcoidosis

Sarcoidosis is a noncaseating granulomatous disease of unclear cause, most commonly involving the lymphatic system, lungs, and skin, although any organ system may be affected. Upper respiratory tract involvement is less common, but the disease may manifest as cervical adenopathy, recurrent sinusitis, epistaxis, and salivary gland infiltration. With nasal involvement, focal areas of hemorrhage, friable mucosa, and discrete yellow submucosal nodules of granulomatous infiltration can be seen on endoscopic examination. Severe nasal infiltration can cause septal perforation or even oronasal fistula. Laryngeal sarcoidosis is a potentially life-threatening manifestation of systemic sarcoidosis that thickens the highly lymphatic supraglottic region. This granulomatous involvement may alter the shape of the epiglottis and result in airway compromise. Unlike GPA, which most commonly affects the subglottis, laryngeal sarcoidosis may rarely cause subglottic stenosis. Symptoms of laryngeal involvement include dysphagia, dyspnea, and hoarseness. Heerfordt syndrome (uveoparotid fever) is a rare manifestation of sarcoidosis presenting with uveitis, parotid swelling, and facial nerve paralysis. Sarcoidosis can also cause masses at the tongue, lips, facial bones, and lacrimal gland presenting as dry eye.

Diagnosis usually involves a biopsy revealing characteristic noncaseating granulomas. Although a definitive serologic diagnostic test does not exist, elevations in angiotensin-converting enzyme with multiorgan system involvement are suggestive of sarcoidosis. Treatment of symptomatic disease typically includes systemic corticosteroids, although some patients may have a benign progression with spontaneous resolution. Nasal symptoms of the disease can be treated using saline irrigation and topical nasal steroids. Select patients may benefit from endoscopic sinus surgery. Localized treatment to maintain airway patency includes intralesional injection of corticosteroids in the case of small well-circumscribed lesions. Obstructive lesions can be excised using carbon dioxide laser or microdebrider in an effort to prevent the need for tracheostomy, although that may be required as a temporary or permanent therapy in severe cases.[3]

### Relapsing polychondritis

A rare inflammatory disorder involving cartilage of the ear, nose, respiratory tract, and joint, relapsing polychondritis (RPC) presents in several ways within the head and neck. Swelling and overlying skin erythema of the auricle sparing the lobule are the most common manifestations. With recurrent inflammatory flares, cartilage may atrophy, and replacement with fibrous connective tissue may cause further cartilaginous destruction, ultimately presenting as ear deformities. The nasal cartilages may also be involved, resulting in crusting and epistaxis, and with chronic inflammation, destruction of the septal cartilage, and saddle nose deformity. In addition to symptoms of chondritis, audiovestibular damage may be present. Chondritis of the airway may manifest as hoarseness, tenderness of the larynx, cough, dyspnea, or stridor. The rigid laryngotracheal structure necessary to maintain airway patency in combination with scarring secondary to recurrent chondritis is a life-threatening manifestation causing airway stenosis and respiratory compromise. Management may be challenging because the larynx, trachea, and even bronchi may lose support and collapse, leading to stenosis.

Diagnosis using the McAdam criteria requires 3 of the following 6 clinical features:

1. Bilateral auricular chondritis
2. Nonerosive, seronegative, inflammatory polyarthritis
3. Nasal chondritis
4. Ocular inflammation
5. Respiratory tract chondritis
6. Cochlear and/or vestibular damage

Laboratory findings reveal nonspecific elevation of inflammatory markers, including erythrocyte sedimentation rate and C-reactive protein. The presence of antinuclear antibody and rheumatoid factor suggests an autoimmune process, and cartilage-specific antibodies may be present during an acute episode of RPC. A biopsy reveals histologic changes consistent with chondritis, chondrolysis, and perichondritis. As with other autoimmune conditions, corticosteroids, and in some cases, immunosuppressive therapy are the mainstay of treatment. Surgical management is used to maintain airway patency, with tracheostomy being a stabilizing option in some.[4]

### Sjögren syndrome

Sjögren syndrome is a chronic autoimmune condition characterized by lymphocytic infiltration and enlargement of the salivary and lacrimal glands producing xerostomia and dry eye, respectively. Sjögren syndrome can present as a primary condition or in association with several autoimmune connective tissue disorders, notably rheumatoid arthritis (RA). In addition to xerostomia, salivary gland involvement can cause cheilitis, dental caries, candidiasis, and dysgeusia. Sjögren syndrome may also present with thyroid abnormalities, dry nasal mucous membrane, recurrent epistaxis, and rarely, sensorineural hearing loss.

Physiologic and iatrogenic causes of xerostomia must be ruled out before a diagnosis of Sjögren syndrome can be applied. Blood tests revealing autoantibodies to Ro (SS-A) and La (SS-B) antigens are strongly suggestive of Sjögren syndrome. Diagnosis is made by biopsy of minor salivary gland cells revealing dense lymphocyte infiltrate. Sjögren syndrome is associated with an increased rate of transformation to B-cell lymphoma, and therefore, these patients require frequent follow-up. Symptomatic treatment uses artificial lubricants for oral and nasal mucosa and artificial tears for dry eyes.[5]

### Amyloidosis

Amyloidosis is an idiopathic condition manifested by the abnormal extracellular deposition of insoluble protein. The most common subtype, AL, is due to an overproduction of normally functioning monoclonal light chains that misfold, aggregate, and ultimately cause tissue damage. There is an association of AL amyloidosis with clonal diseases, including multiple myeloma. Common head and neck manifestations of amyloidosis include periorbital purpura and macroglossia. The latter may be subtle and asymptomatic or severe enough to alter voice, swallowing, or even breathing in extreme cases. Laryngeal amyloidosis most commonly represents an isolated form of amyloidosis but can rarely present with systemic disease or multiple myeloma. Involvement of the larynx localizes to the cords, manifesting as hoarseness, cough, dyspnea, or stridor.[6]

Diagnosis is classically made via a biopsy with Congo red staining demonstrating bright green birefringence under polarizing light microscopy. If amyloidosis is diagnosed on biopsy, a systemic workup should be done to assess further organ involvement. The therapeutic goal in laryngeal amyloidosis is the maintenance of airway patency and management of voice quality, which can be achieved using suspension microlaryngoscopy to excise involved tissues. Rarely, surgical debulking of lingual amyloidosis may be necessary.[4]

### Systemic lupus erythematosus

Systemic lupus erythematosus (SLE) is an autoimmune condition affecting multiple organ systems. SLE classically presents with fever, rash, and joint pain. Common head and neck manifestations of SLE include the characteristic malar rash and ulcerations of the nasal and oral mucosa. Histopathologic diagnosis of mucosal lesions reveals immunoglobulins and complements along the basement membrane of the dermal-epidermal junction. This biopsy is important to differentiate mucosal ulcerations of SLE from other causes, including lichen planus or leukoplakia.

### Rheumatoid arthritis

RA is a chronic inflammatory disorder primarily affecting the joints and is capable of head and neck manifestations involving the temporomandibular joint (TMJ) and cricoarytenoid joints of the larynx. TMJ involvement presents as locking, crepitus, and tenderness to palpation, all of which worsen with mastication. Acute laryngeal involvement appears as tenderness and erythema on laryngoscopic examination and presents clinically with hoarseness. Progression to chronic ankylosis can lead to airway impairment secondary to reduced vocal fold mobility. Given the fixation of the joints in a partially adducted position, this can pose a challenge to intubation. Extraarticular manifestations of the head and neck include submucosal nodules of the vocal fold ("bamboo nodules") similar to the cutaneous rheumatoid nodules. Therapy for cricoarytenoid involvement may include intra-articular steroid injection. Surgery to maintain a glottis airway may be needed in severe or recalcitrant cases, including cordotomy, arytenoidectomy, or tracheostomy. Vocal fold rheumatoid nodules can be treated using intralesional steroid injection or microsurgical resection.[4]

### Kawasaki disease

Kawasaki disease is a rare medium vessel granulomatous disease celebrated for affecting the coronary arteries supplying the heart. Generally self-limiting, Kawasaki disease classically presents with conjunctivitis sparing the limbus, cervical lymphadenopathy, an erythematous, desquamating rash on the palms of the hands and soles of the feet, and a swollen, "strawberry tongue" in a young patient with high fever. Treatment consists of high-dose aspirin and immunoglobulins in an effort to reduce fever and inflammation. Typically, treatment results in a full recovery and prevents progression to the coronary artery involvement.

### Behçet disease

A unique type of vasculitis affecting both arterial and venous vessels, Behçet disease is characterized by inflammation of the oral cavity, genitals, and eyes. The common presentation includes recurrent oral ulcers that are typically larger, longer lasting, and more painful than aphthous ulcers. Ulcers may also extend into the nasal cavity to cause symptoms of rhinorrhea and pain. Diagnosis is made clinically; however, the presence of pathergy, or slowed healing, is strongly indicative of Behçet disease.[4]

### Giant cell arteritis

Giant cell arteritis (GCA) is a large vessel granulomatous disease that primarily affects branches of the external carotid artery. Dependent upon location, GCA can present with headache if the superficial temporal artery is implicated, visual changes if the ophthalmic artery is implicated, or claudication with mastication if the facial artery is involved. Diagnosis relies on segmental arterial biopsy to reveal giant cells. Because areas of the vessel may be unaffected, a negative result does not fully rule out GCA. Therapy includes systemic steroids, which should be started before receiving biopsy, if there is strong clinical suspicion in an effort to reduce the risk of vision loss.

## Cutaneous Disease

### Pemphigus vulgaris

An autoimmune condition characterized by mucocutaneous blistering, pemphigus vulgaris affects the epidermal-dermal junction to form cutaneous and mucosal blebs. Lesions appear as thin, round bullae primarily in areas of friction. These lesions easily rupture, leaving a hemorrhagic crust that heals slowly and poses difficulty for diagnosis. The oral cavity is the most common site of mucosal lesions and may be the only manifestation of pemphigus vulgaris. These painful lesions, primarily present on the buccal mucosa and gingiva, worsen with mastication, and erode quickly, leading to bleeding and extreme salivation. Lesions can also present in the nasal mucosa, even extending to the larynx and esophagus to produce symptoms of dysphagia, hoarseness, progressive stridor, and dyspnea. Nikolsky sign, or the blistering of normal skin or mucosa with mechanical pressure, is positive in patients with pemphigus vulgaris, and patients often have immunoglobulin G autoantibodies to desmoglein 1 and desmoglein 3. Definitive diagnosis is made using a tissue biopsy revealing intraepithelial acantholysis. Systemic glucocorticoids are the primary treatment, although food avoidance and oral hygiene can effectively decrease oral symptoms.

### Pemphigoid

Pemphigoid is an uncommon autoimmune condition characterized by subepithelial blistering. Clinically distinct from pemphigus by the lack of acantholysis, pemphigoid is commonly classified into 2 subtypes, bullous and cicatricial. Bullous pemphigoid presents as acute pruritic blistering of the skin that often heals without scarring. Although bullous pemphigoid can spread to the buccal mucosa, this is less common than the oral ulcerations that present in cicatricial pemphigoid. Unlike bullous pemphigoid, the lesions of cicatricial pemphigoid tend to scar, which may result in functional impairment, including vision loss, hoarseness, dysphagia, or airway compromise. Direct immunofluorescence of biopsy specimen reveals characteristic antibodies at the basement membrane.

### Lichen planus

Lichen planus is a chronic, mucocutaneous autoimmune condition that can commonly involves the oral cavity, most often the buccal mucosa, tongue, and gingiva. Primarily appearing as white, reticular patterned asymptomatic lesions, lichen planus can also present as erythematous or erosive disease causing sensations of burning and pain. The primary goal of treatment is the reduction of pain and inflammation, usually achieved through the use of topical immunosuppressants. Because of the possible malignant transformation, patients with lichen planus, particularly those with erosions, should be followed closely.[7]

### Mucociliary Disease

### Cystic fibrosis

Cystic fibrosis (CF) is an autosomal recessive condition caused by various mutations of the CF gene coding for CF transmembrane conductance regulator (CFTR) protein. Despite normally functioning cilia, dysfunctional CFTR protein leads to thickened secretions that make mucociliary transport difficult. The hallmarks of CF include chronic lung disease, chronic sinusitis, pancreatic insufficiency, and a history of meconium ileus at birth. Recurrent rhinosinusitis in CF patients presents with thickened rhinorrhea, nasal obstruction, and ultimately, nasal polyps. In children presenting with nasal polyps, clinical suspicion for CF should be heightened. Chronic rhinosinusitis may also lead to some underdevelopment of the paranasal sinuses, particularly the frontal sinuses, although all sinuses may show signs of hypoplasia. Some patients will not present with active symptoms of chronic rhinosinusitis but may still have positive findings on CT imaging.

Diagnosis of CF is confirmed using the sweat chloride test as well as genetic testing. The treatment goals from an otolaryngologic perspective in CF are to maintain a patent nasal airway and minimize infection. Primary treatment includes nasal irrigation, steroids, and antibiotics. Surgical intervention, such as endoscopic sinus surgery, may be considered to remove polyps or enlarge sinus openings in order to improve secretion management and reduce stagnation. Sinonasal disease may have a negative impact on pulmonary disease, and therefore, multidisciplinary approaches in management must be emphasized.

### Primary ciliary dyskinesia
Primary ciliary dyskinesia is a disorder characterized by chronic respiratory tract infection and infertility, due to a loss of ultrastructural ciliary components despite the presence of morphologically intact cilia. This deficiency alters the mobility of the cilia and leads to ineffective mucociliary transport, thus producing stagnation of secretions, which increases the frequency of infection. Manifestations of the head and neck present in childhood as chronic rhinosinusitis, cough, and otitis media. Diagnosis is made via biopsy of the respiratory mucosa at the inferior turbinate or carina and investigation under electron microscopy for ultrastructural defects. Symptomatic treatment includes antibiotics to prevent infection and the use of nasal irrigation. Surgical intervention can include endoscopic sinus surgery to improve sinus drainage pattern in patients with recurrent infections. Pulmonary therapies, similar to those used with CF, are often used to reduce pulmonary infections.

### Infectious Disease

### Virus
**Human papillomavirus** Infection with the human papillomavirus (HPV), a double-stranded DNA virus, is common and often asymptomatic. If persistent, HPV can lead to papilloma or precancerous lesions. HPV types 6 and 11 are most responsible for warts, including papillomatosis of the nose, oropharynx, and larynx. Laryngeal papillomatosis (recurrent respiratory papillomatosis) may present with chronic hoarseness in adults, and rarely, dyspnea. In children, this can be both an airway and voice issue. In both cases, although not curative of the infection, surgical intervention is warranted to improve voice and maintain airway patency. Diagnosis of HPV infection is made using in situ hybridization or polymerase chain reaction.

Well known for its relationship with cervical cancer, infection with HPV-16 (and much less commonly -18, -31, and -33) has been recently associated with an increasing number of oropharyngeal squamous cell carcinomas, including the base of tongue and tonsils. The growing number of HPV-related oropharyngeal cancers is presenting in a younger population and is associated with sexual risk factors. Unlike non-HPV-related oropharyngeal cancers, these carcinomas are independent of alcohol or tobacco use.[8]

**Herpes simplex virus type 1** Herpes simplex virus type 1 (HSV-1) is a double-stranded DNA virus causing a common, lifelong infection that is primarily asymptomatic but can produce bouts of painful, self-limited lesions of the oral cavity, known as cold sores. Primary infection occurs by viral invasion of the mucus membrane causing oral lesions in addition to gingivostomatitis and pharyngitis. The virus can then travel via the sensory nerve endings to the sensory ganglia, where it remains latent until reactivation occurs. HSV-1 can rarely infect the eye, causing symptoms of pain, blurry vision, and discharge, or the airway, to cause epiglottitis or laryngitis. Treatment can include acyclovir.

HSV-1 reactivation has become widely accepted as a cause of Bell palsy, a sudden onset unilateral facial palsy affecting the seventh cranial nerve without known other cause (eg, neoplasm, trauma). Bell palsy presents as brow ptosis, inability to close the eye, and loss of the nasolabial fold. The treatment of Bell palsy secondary to infection with HSV-1 includes oral glucocorticoids and acyclovir therapy. Treatment can improve recovery rates, and in combination with good moisturizing eye care, minimize complications secondary to incomplete eyelid closure.[9]

**Varicella-zoster virus** Infection with the varicella-zoster virus (VZV) can produce vesicles of the upper respiratory mucus membranes in children. Cutaneous lesions exist on a progressive scale and persist simultaneously in various stages ranging from new eruptions to crusted vesicles. A rare but painful reactivation of VZV is responsible for Ramsay Hunt syndrome (herpes zoster oticus). Lesions can present on the auricle, ear canal, and tympanic membrane. VZV is also implicated as a causative agent in Bell palsy, contrasted from HSV cause by the external vesicles and pain. In addition to facial nerve palsy, the first division of the trigeminal nerve can be involved, causing unilateral pain and vesicles on the face and oral cavity. Treatment with prednisone and acyclovir is recommended.

**Epstein-Barr virus** Infection with the Epstein-Barr virus (EBV) typically causes infectious mononucleosis. Also referred to as "glandular fever," infectious mononucleosis is characterized by lymphadenopathy, fever, and tonsillar pharyngitis. Lymph node involvement is commonly bilaterally at the posterior and jugular cervical nodes. Tonsillar involvement may involve gray exudate and may rarely progress to peritonsillar abscess or even occlusion of the airway. Laboratory findings show elevated lymphocytes, and histology of the lymph node may reveal Reed-Sternberg cells. The head and neck manifestations are generally self-limited.

**Mumps virus** Mumps is caused by an RNA paramyxovirus. Commonly affecting children, mumps manifests as swelling of the parotid and salivary glands. Considered a vaccine-preventable disease, mumps infection can lead to complications, including sensorineural hearing loss, vestibular symptoms, and thyroiditis. Diagnosis can be confirmed using immunoglobulin antibody testing.

### Bacteria
**Mycobacterium tuberculosis** Tuberculosis (TB) is a major global health problem that is caused by the bacterium *Mycobacterium tuberculosis*. Primarily affecting the lungs, TB involvement of the cervical and submandibular lymph nodes can present as a chronic, painless cervical adenopathy called scrofula. Laryngeal TB was formerly thought to be caused by clumps of bacilli coughed up from the lungs during active pulmonary infection but is now theorized to be the result of hematologic or lymphatic spread in immunocompromised patients. Laryngeal TB lesions, potentially mistaken as cancer on examination, appear as nodular, ulcerated interarytenoid lesions, which cause hoarseness, dysphagia, cough, and weight loss. TB lesions may also present as nasal or oral mucosal lesions, and in the middle ear may produce clear, odorless otorrhea, and hearing loss. Biopsied lesions show caseating granulomas and mycobacterial organisms, with other diagnostic techniques including sputum culture and chest radiograph potentially helpful to confirm the diagnosis. Effective treatment of TB is difficult because of the bacterial composition; however, maintenance includes a combination of antibiotic therapies.[10]

**Atypical mycobacterium** A variety of infectious pathogens, including the *Mycobacterium avium* complex (MAC) and *Mycobacterium scrofulaceum*, can cause atypical mycobacterium infection. Known to infect children and immunocompromised patients, infection with atypical mycobacterium manifests as firm, painless cervicofacial lymphadenitis, commonly in the submandibular region. Rarely presenting with constitutional or pulmonary symptoms, infection with atypical mycobacterium is important to distinguish from TB. This distinction can be made using clinical presentation, blood culture, and imaging, because the treatment options differ. Because of resistance to medical therapy, lymph nodes are often treated by complete surgical excision.[10]

**Treponema pallidum** Syphilis is caused by infection with the bacteria *Treponema pallidum* and classically presents in a series of 4 progressive stages. The primary stage consists of a painless chancre, whereas secondary syphilis produces a diffuse rash involving the skin and mucous membranes. The third stage is a latent, asymptomatic stage lasting for years before final progression to tertiary syphilis characterized by gummas, which may perforate the nasal septum or palate to create oronasal fistulae. Congenital syphilis transmitted to the neonate may present as mucoid rhinorrhea, perioral scarring radiating from the vermilion border, saddle nose, and "Hutchinson's teeth," described as notched, hypoplastic, and lacking enamel. Otosyphilis as a cause of sensorineural hearing loss has been previously proposed, although a clear pathogenic mechanism has yet to be described. Diagnosis can be made using treponemal blood tests, and classic treatment of syphilis is penicillin.[11]

**Actinomyces israelii** Actinomycosis is caused by infection with *Actinomyces israelii*, a microaerophilic gram-positive organism normally present in the oral cavity but increasing to infectious levels in the presence of dental caries, periodontal disease, or trauma. Infection produces suppurative granulomas of the oral cavity, cervical adenitis, and purulent drainage from sinus tracts. Most infected patients present with cervicofacial actinomycosis; however, cases of laryngeal and tracheal involvement have been reported. Diagnosis can be difficult, but characteristic sulfur granules with a "sunburst" appearance are seen in the purulent discharge. Antibiotic treatment primarily consists of prolonged administration of penicillin.[4]

*Fungus*
**Candida albicans** Candidiasis is caused by overgrowth of *Candida albicans*, a fungus normally present within the digestive tract, skin, and mucus membranes. Candidiasis infection of the oropharynx and oral cavity, "thrush," presents with white pseudomembranous patches, erythema, mucosal atrophy, loss of taste, and pain. Candidiasis can also affect the external auditory meatus, larynx, and esophagus. Patients are typically immunocompromised, but infection can also be due to endocrine disorders, nutritional deficiencies, poor oral hygiene, the use of steroid inhalers, and systemic steroids.[12]

**Others** Numerous fungi species can cause focal head and neck manifestations, including histoplasmosis, blastomycosis, crytococcosis, and coccidiomycosis. Laryngeal involvement, often coincident with pulmonary disease, may cause hoarseness, dysphagia, odynophagia, or upper airway compromise. Oral mucosal involvement may present as nodular lesions or ulceration. Skin and lymph nodes may also be involved.[12]

### Disorders of Immunodeficiency and Malignancy

#### Acquired immunodeficiency syndrome
AIDS is characterized by the presence of opportunistic disease in a patient infected with the human immunodeficiency virus (HIV). HIV attacks immune cells, leading to a decrease in $CD4^+$ T cells, which places the patient at risk for infection with opportunistic organisms, such as in candidiasis. Recurrent rhinosinusitis, otitis media, and pharyngitis may occur in patients with AIDS, and noncancerous oropharyngeal ulcerations may also be present because of several infectious causes. In addition,

neoplastic lesions, such as Kaposi sarcoma, may manifest as oral discomfort, even extending to the nasopharynx or larynx, with persistent unexplained cervical adenopathy and purple palatal lesions. Cervical lymphadenopathy and hypertrophy along the Waldeyer ring of lymphoid tissue are common in AIDS patients. Lymphoepithelial cysts in salivary glands, particularly the parotid gland, can be an early and pathognomonic sign of HIV infection. Diagnosis of HIV infection may be made using enzyme-linked immunosorbent assay to detect antibodies, and the presence of viral proteins is confirmed using Western blot.[13]

### Polymorphic reticulosis
Polymorphic reticulosis, also known as midline malignant reticulosis, is a precursor T-cell proliferation of the nose that can mimic acute unilateral sinusitis at onset. Polymorphic reticulosis presents with nasal obstruction, purulent rhinorrhea, and serosanguinous discharge, and progression of this T-cell lymphoma can lead to mucosal ulceration, appearing pale and friable, and may extend beyond the nose to the palate, maxillary sinus, and upper lip. As with any ulceration involving the nasal cavity, severe lesions can cause septal perforation or even oronasal fistulae. Polymorphic lymphoid infiltrate is characterized by an angiocentric pattern and is capable of invading the vessels, leading to infarction and necrosis. A role for EBV infection in the cause of polymorphic reticulosis has been proposed but has yet to be definitively determined.[14]

## Vascular Disorders

### Hereditary hemorrhagic telangiectasia
Hereditary hemorrhagic telangiectasia, also known by the eponym Osler-Weber-Rendu syndrome, is an autosomal dominant disorder of the skin and vasculature causing abnormal vessel formation. Telangiectasias of the nasal mucosa are responsible for chronic epistaxis, and those of the skin and mouth are less problematic but can be cosmetically displeasing. Ulceration may sometimes occur. Management of the recurrent epistaxis may include laser ablation of the telangiectasias, cautery, or septodermoplasty.

## Metabolic Disorders

### Diabetes mellitus
A rare but severe otolaryngologic complication of diabetes is acute necrotizing otitis externa (malignant otitis externa). This infection causes purulent otorrhea, edema of the ear canal, and severe deep-seated otalgia secondary to insignificant trauma. On clinical observation, cartilaginous necrosis, external auditory canal granulation, and exposed bone can be diagnostic of this complication. Periodontal disease is also associated with poorly controlled diabetes. Furthermore, diabetes predisposes patients to peripheral neuropathies, which can impair the sensations of taste and smell.

## Bone Disorders

### Fibrous dysplasia
Because of a mutation of the guanine nucleotide stimulatory protein (GNAS1), fibrous dysplasia causes portions of normal bone to be replaced by fibrous connective tissue. Many patients are asymptomatic, but the disease can cause pain and swelling and places patients at an increased fracture risk. Behaving as a slow-growing mass lesion, the involvement of facial bones can distort surrounding structures, including the facial nerve, nasal airway, middle ear ossicles, and teeth. Compression of the optic nerve, globe, ossicles, and nasal airway is common with rapid expansion, and surgical resection is indicated in these patients.

### Osteogenesis imperfecta

Osteogenesis imperfecta (OI) is an inherited connective tissue condition affecting cartilage development due to mutations in the alpha-1 or alpha-2 chains of type 1 collagen. Also called "brittle bone disease" for its phenotypic presentation, OI classically manifests as multiple fractures associated with little traumatic force. In addition to short stature and easy bruising, the disease presents clinically with head and neck manifestations, including basilar skull deformities, blue sclerae, hearing loss, and dentinogenesis imperfecta. Hearing loss is also common in OI, but usually is not detected clinically until adolescence or adulthood. Thus, patients with OI should be monitored regularly for both sensorineural and conductive hearing loss.

### Neurologic Disorders

### Myasthenia gravis

Myasthenia gravis (MG) is an autoimmune condition affecting the neuromuscular junction. Caused by antibodies against acetylcholine receptors, MG leads to episodic and progressive muscle weakness that improves with rest. Initially, MG classically presents with ptosis, and other manifestations within the head and neck include dysphagia, velopharyngeal insufficiency, dysarthria, dyspnea, and generalized facial weakness, including the "hanging jaw sign." The disease can be managed medically, and symptomatic therapy can be used if the ability to breathe is compromised.

### Amyotrophic lateral sclerosis

Amyotrophic lateral sclerosis (ALS) classically involves both upper and lower motor neurons to cause progressive muscle weakness, incoordination, atrophy, and

---

**Box 1**
**Systemic causes of oral ulcerations**

Granulomatosis with polyangiitis

Eosinophilic granulomatosis with polyangiitis

Systemic lupus erythematosus

Behçet disease

Pemphigus vulgaris

Cicatricial pemphigoid

Lichen planus

Herpes simplex virus-1

Varicella-zoster virus

Epstein-Barr virus

Syphilis

Fungal infection

Linear immunoglobulin A disease

Erythema multiforme

Tuberculosis

Cyclic neutropenia

Hereditary hemorrhagic telangiectasia

fasciculations. Bulbar ALS describes a presentation of ALS involving the cranial nerves. This presentation may represent an isolated form, although more commonly is a bulbar onset before a generalized presentation of ALS. Patients with bulbar ALS present with dysphagia, spastic dysarthria, and pseudobulbar affect, the inappropriate response such as yawning, laughing, or crying to a stimulus. Patients may experience laryngospasm impairing inspiration and speech for brief periods of time. Bulbar dysfunction is responsible for decreased tone in the muscles of mastication leading to difficulty opening the mouth, or trismus. Other manifestations of bulbar ALS include tongue fasciculations, incomplete eye closure, difficulty chewing, and drooling. Diagnosis is primarily clinical, based on history and examination findings, although it may also be supported with electrodiagnostic studies.

## FUTURE CONSIDERATIONS/SUMMARY

The manifestations of systemic disease in the head and neck region are important for Internists and Otolaryngologists alike. The presentations of many of these disorders overlap, but with careful evaluation, additional diagnostic testing, and astute clinical acumen, these systemic diseases can be identified. Several of these disorders may create urgent, and particularly with the airway involvement, even emergent situations. Careful monitoring in those patients with diagnosed systemic disorders can improve the timely involvement of otolaryngology–head and neck surgeons to prevent complications and minimize morbidity and potential mortality from such. Many of these processes require a multidisciplinary approach, including internal medicine providers, otolaryngologists, rheumatologists, dentists and oral surgeons, infectious disease specialists, pulmonologists, pathologists, and radiologists. This article has reviewed select systemic diseases and infections but cannot be all inclusive in this limited format. To aid in evaluation and management of these patients, 2 boxes are provided. **Box 1** represents a differential diagnosis for oral ulceration, a common manifestation of several disorders. Conditions with the potential for airway compromise may require urgent consultation of the otolaryngologist and are presented in **Box 2** as reference.

---

**Box 2**
**Systemic disease with the potential for airway compromise**

Granulomatosis with polyangiitis

Sarcoidosis

Relapsing polychondritis

Amyloidosis

Rheumatoid arthritis

Cicatricial pemphigoid

Human papillomavirus

Tuberculosis

Fungal infection

Myasthenia gravis

Amyotrophic lateral sclerosis

Angioedema

## REFERENCES

1. Gubbels SP, Barkhuizen A, Hwang PH. Head and neck manifestations of Wegener's granulomatosis. Otolaryngol Clin North Am 2003;36(4):685–705.
2. Greco A, Rizzo MI, De Virgilio A, et al. Churg–Strauss syndrome. Autoimmun Rev 2015;14(4):341–8.
3. Schwartzbauer HR, Tami TA. Ear, nose, and throat manifestations of sarcoidosis. Otolaryngol Clin North Am 2003;36(4):673–84.
4. Flint P. Cummings otolaryngology–head & neck surgery. 6th edition. Philadelphia: Elsevier/Saunders; 2015. p. 176–226.
5. Mahoney EJ, Spiegel JH. Sjögren's disease. Otolaryngol Clin North Am 2003; 36(4):733–45.
6. Hazenberg BPC. Amyloidosis: a clinical overview. Rheum Dis Clin North Am 2013;39(2):323–45.
7. Gonzalez-Moles MA, Scully C, Gil-Montoya JA. Oral lichen planus: controversies surrounding malignant transformation. Oral Dis 2008;14(3):229–43.
8. Spence T, Bruce J, Yip KW, et al. HPV associated head and neck cancer. Cancers (Basel) 2016;8(8) [pii:E75].
9. Kennedy PG. Herpes simplex virus type 1 and Bell's palsy-a current assessment of the controversy. J Neurovirol 2010;16(1):1–5.
10. Munck K, Mandpe AH. Mycobacterial infections of the head and neck. Otolaryngol Clin North Am 2003;36(4):569–76.
11. Pletcher SD, Cheung SW. Syphilis and otolaryngology. Otolaryngol Clin North Am 2003;36(4):595–605, vi.
12. Thrasher RD, Kingdom TT. Fungal infections of the head and neck: an update. Otolaryngol Clin North Am 2003;36(4):577–94.
13. Gurney TA, Murr AH. Otolaryngologic manifestations of human immunodeficiency virus infection. Otolaryngol Clin North Am 2003;36(4):607–24.
14. Van Gorp J, Weiping L, Jacobse K, et al. Epstein-Barr virus in nasal T-cell lymphomas (polymorphic reticulosis/midline malignant reticulosis) in Western China. J Pathol 1994;173(2):81–7.

# Urgent Infections of the Head and Neck

Marika D. Russell, MD*, Matthew S. Russell, MD

## KEYWORDS

- Sinusitis • Mastoiditis • Peritonsillar abscess • Urgent • Airway

## KEY POINTS

- Infection of the head and neck is common and, in most cases, may be appropriately managed by the primary care provider. However, some infections can be associated with significant morbidity and timely recognition is critical.
- Deep neck space infections originating in the oral cavity, pharynx, or salivary glands may be complicated by airway or mediastinal involvement.
- Otologic infection can be complicated by spread within the skull base or intracranial cavity.
- Complications of sinusitis may include spread of infection to the orbit or brain.
- Invasive fungal sinusitis is a rare but devastating disease that requires a high index of suspicion to diagnose and treat effectively.

## INTRODUCTION

Infection occurs commonly in the head and neck. In 2016, 11% of the US adult population was diagnosed with sinusitis.[1] In children, acute otitis media is a leading cause of visits to a health care provider,[2] and sore throat accounts for 2.1% of ambulatory visits in the United States.[3] For an overwhelming number of cases, management of uncomplicated head and neck infections by the primary care provider is appropriate. Yet, because of the anatomic proximity of common infectious sites to the orbit and brain, and because of the potential for involvement of the upper airway and mediastinum, infections of the head and neck can be associated with significant clinical morbidity or mortality. It is these instances in which timely recognition of the clinical problem is imperative and involvement of specialty expertise is warranted. Often, the treatment of complicated infections of the head and neck requires multidisciplinary management. The primary goal of this article is to enable the primary care provider to recognize these clinical presentations so that timely facilitation of treatment may occur.

Disclosure Statement: The authors have no financial disclosures to make.
Otolaryngology–Head and Neck Surgery, University of California, San Francisco, 2233 Post Street, 3rd floor, San Francisco, CA 94115, USA
* Corresponding author. 1001 Potrero Avenue, 3A, San Francisco, CA 94110.
*E-mail address:* marika.russell@ucsf.edu

Patients at increased risk for complicated head and neck infection include those with diabetes, immune compromise, and advanced age. Diabetic patients, in particular, have been shown to have increased risk of suppuration, multispace infections, and a need for multiple surgical procedures.[4] Delay in surgical treatment of head and neck abscesses is associated with increased risk of complications and prolonged hospital stay.[5] Timely recognition of clinical conditions requiring urgent management is especially important in these groups.

## DEEP NECK SPACE INFECTIONS

Infections involving the oral cavity, oropharynx, and salivary glands are common. Approximately 30% of deep neck space infections are associated with an odontogenic source, 30% are associated with pharyngitis, and 10% develop in the setting of sialadenitis.[6] Less common causes of deep neck infection include suppurative lymphadenitis, infection of congenital cysts, otologic infection, and injection drug use.

Complications of infection occur when infection spreads beyond the primary site of origin. Initially, this involves cellulitis or abscess formation adjacent to the site of infection. If not addressed promptly, infection may spread from the originating site to the deep neck spaces bounded by fascial planes. These spaces most commonly include the submandibular triangle, parapharyngeal or retropharyngeal space, and masticator space. Urgent evaluation and management of deep space neck infections is imperative because progression may result in airway compromise, either through direct mass effect or local edema. Additionally, spread of infection to the tissues of the mediastinum can have devastating consequences, including mediastinitis and development of pleural and pericardial effusion or empyema. Mediastinal extension of infection is associated with mortality rates of up to 40%.[7]

### Oral Cavity and Salivary Glands

In the oral cavity, odontogenic infection arises from the tooth or its supporting structures and often resolves if prompt treatment of the infectious source is undertaken.[8] Similarly, sialadenitis may arise from salivary stasis in the setting of dehydration or sialolithiasis and responds to treatment with oral antibiotics, hydration measures, and use of sialagogues to encourage salivary flow. However, progression of odontogenic or submandibular gland infection can lead to serious complications, including Ludwig angina, which requires urgent intervention.

Ludwig angina is an infection in the floor of mouth space contained by the mylohyoid muscle and is characterized by prominent rapid swelling in the floor of mouth due to edema, cellulitis, or abscess formation. Swelling is marked, such that the submandibular papillae on the floor of mouth can be observed protruding above the level of the lower incisors (**Fig. 1**). This results in relative macroglossia, with displacement of the tongue posteriorly. Posterior glossoptosis may lead to significant airway obstruction at the oropharyngeal level. Airway management in this setting is challenging, and timely and appropriate intervention is paramount. Because of obstruction generated at the level of the oropharynx, mask ventilation or oral intubation may not be possible. Instead, the airway must be secured with the patient spontaneously breathing via awake fiberoptic intubation or awake tracheotomy. Attempts to manipulate the tissues of the oral cavity and oropharynx for the purposes of oral intubation may provoke rapid worsening of edema and should be avoided.

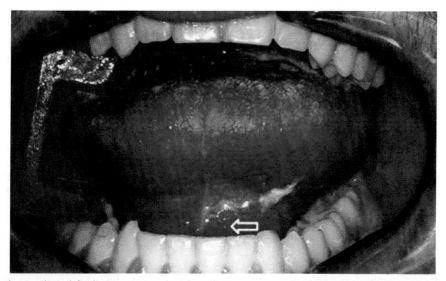

**Fig. 1.** Clinical findings associated with Ludwig angina. Note the superior floor of mouth displacement with elevation of the submandibular papillae (*arrow*) above the level of the lower incisors.

### Oropharynx

In the oropharynx, untreated bacterial tonsillitis may progress to peritonsillar abscess (PTA). A typical clinical course for PTA includes 3 to 5 days of sore throat, followed by unilateral worsening of pain, and is often accompanied by ipsilateral otalgia. Patients may present with fever, dysphagia, trismus, and so-called hot potato voice. On examination, unilateral palatal effacement, or bulging of the palate, is the typical finding (**Fig. 2**). Uvular deviation, often described as a feature of PTA, is poorly specific and

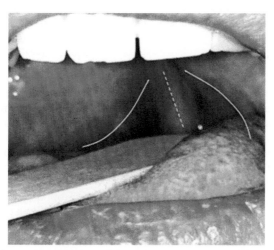

**Fig. 2.** Right sided PTA. Note bulging of the right palate relative to the left (*solid line*). The uvular axis is deviated (*dotted line*).

should not be considered a diagnostic finding in and of itself. Typically, infection occurs at the superior pole of the tonsil, which results in effacement and bulging of the soft palate. Diagnosis can, therefore, be made by clinical examination without the need for additional imaging in most cases. Less commonly, infection occurs at the inferior pole, which can lead to the appearance of tonsillar asymmetry but the abscess may otherwise not be readily clinically apparent. Unilateral tonsillar asymmetry should prompt otolaryngology evaluation due to the possibility of occult abscesses or neoplasm.

The management of PTA requires drainage of the abscess either by needle aspiration or incision and drainage. The choice of technique is outside the scope of this article; however, both are considered acceptable clinical practice if performed appropriately.[9] If not recognized in a timely fashion, parapharyngeal or retropharyngeal extension can occur, which may lead to the development of laryngeal edema and airway compromise. In particular, PTAs of the inferior pole may be associated with epiglottitis and require prompt evaluation and management.[10]

### Emergent Neck Infections

Lemierre syndrome is a rare complication of head and neck infection. Classic features include suppurative thrombophlebitis of the internal jugular vein with production of septic thromboemboli to the lungs. In the preantibiotic era, this clinical condition was almost uniformly fatal; however, modern imaging techniques and early (often incidental) diagnosis allows for prompt treatment, including surgical drainage of the primary infectious site, anticoagulation, and intravenous antibiotic therapy. If addressed promptly, complete recovery may be achieved in most cases.[11]

Necrotizing skin and soft tissue infections of the head and neck are also uncommon but require urgent recognition and intervention. Treatment includes broad-spectrum antibiotics and wide surgical debridement. Odontogenic infection underlies most cases, present in up to 80%.[12] Infection is often mixed aerobic and anaerobic, and can involve varying layers of the skin and soft tissue, from skin and subcutaneous lymphatics to deep muscle groups.[13,14] Early signs of infection include erythema or skin discoloration, which can progress to skin darkening and necrosis. Crepitus is often present and soft tissue emphysema can be observed on computed tomography (CT) imaging. If left untreated, necrotizing soft tissue infections can progress rapidly to shock and multiorgan system failure, with mortality rates of 22% to 100%.[14]

## OTOLOGIC INFECTION

Complications of acute otitis media occur with far less morbidity than in the preantibiotic era but nonetheless require urgent recognition and treatment. Infection of the middle ear space may progress directly through suppurative bony destruction or through thrombophlebitic spread. Key features of complicated otologic infection that should be recognized include facial nerve paresis or paralysis, meningeal involvement, and suppuration extending beyond the local confines of the middle ear and mastoid space. These findings should prompt evaluation with a CT scan, which should be performed with intravenous contrast administration.

### Acute Mastoiditis

Acute mastoiditis is the most common complication of suppurative otitis media and is most often seen in children.[15] Acute mastoiditis represents a destructive bacterial infection of the mastoid bone with coalescence of its air cell spaces. Importantly, acute clinical mastoiditis should be differentiated from radiologic mastoiditis, which relates a radiologic finding of fluid (infectious or otherwise) in the mastoid air spaces without the destruction of bony septae. Radiologic observation of fluid opacification in the mastoid space without evidence of acute mastoiditis should be interpreted in the context of the patient's clinical condition and does not necessarily require intervention.

Key features associated with the development of acute mastoiditis include a recent history of clinically apparent acute otitis media (in approximately half of patients), fever, and pain. Examination findings may include abnormal appearance of the tympanic membrane or external auditory canal, postauricular edema and erythema, and protrusion or proptosis of the auricle.[15]

Treatment of acute mastoiditis should, at a minimum, involve culture-directed intravenous antibiotic therapy. Common pathogens include *Streptococcus pneumoniae*, *Pseudomonas aeruginosa*, and *Staphylococcus aureus*.[16] The indications and timing of surgical treatment are outside the scope of this review but may include placement of a tympanostomy tube or mastoidectomy. The goals of surgery are to drain the infection and retrieve purulent fluid for culture.

### Extracranial Complications of Otologic Infection

Acute mastoiditis itself may be complicated by spread of infection outside the middle ear and mastoid space. This occurs through local bony destruction and direct bacterial invasion, or through thrombophlebitic spread. Although fortunately uncommon, complications of mastoiditis can be life-threatening and require prompt recognition and intervention.

Suppuration within the mastoid cavity may extend through the mastoid cortex with development of a subperiosteal abscess, the most common complication of mastoiditis. Seen more commonly in children, subperiosteal abscess presents with erythema and fluctuance in the postauricular region, often with proptosis or protrusion of the auricle. Varied surgical treatment algorithms have been proposed, though incision and drainage of the subperiosteal abscess is required at a minimum.[17]

Suppuration within the mastoid cavity may also erupt through the mastoid tip, extending into the neck along the digastric and sternocleidomastoid muscles, with subsequent formation of a neck abscess. This has been termed Bezold abscess, after the German otologist who described this complication. Presenting features may include neck pain and swelling, which accompany the otologic findings seen in mastoiditis. Although subperiosteal abscess in children is still observed, Bezold abscess is rare in children because it requires aeration of the mastoid tip, which is uncommon in this age group.[18]

Rarely, suppuration may erupt anteriorly toward the root of the zygoma, extending beneath the periosteum of the temporalis muscle. Also described by Bezold,[18] this presents as a facial abscess and is exceedingly uncommon (**Fig. 3**).

Another recognized complication of suppurative mastoiditis results from propagation of suppuration to the petrous apex with subsequent involvement of adjacent cranial nerves V and VI. Gradenigo syndrome describes a classic triad of suppurative otitis media, abducens palsy, and pain in the distribution of the trigeminal nerve.

Finally, it should be noted that presence of cholesteatoma presents a unique precondition for complicated mastoiditis. Cholesteatoma is a chronic process characterized by entrapment of squamous debris within the middle ear and mastoid, with bony erosion occurring over time. If bacterial superinfection within the middle ear and mastoid develops, structures normally covered by bone, including the facial nerve and vestibular labyrinth, may be at increased risk for involvement. Symptoms of suppurative labyrinthitis include profound unilateral hearing loss and vertigo with ataxia,

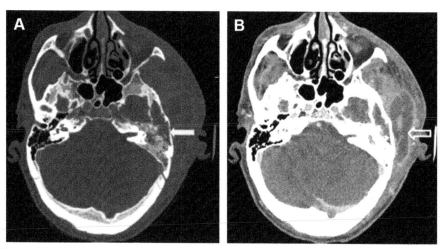

**Fig. 3.** Coalescent mastoiditis with soft tissue abscess. (*A*) In this axial CT with contrast, bone window demonstrates loss of bony septations within the mastoid cavity (*closed arrow*). (*B*) Soft tissue window demonstrates an associated rim-enhancing fluid collection (*open arrow*).

nausea, and vomiting. Patients suspected of having suppurative labyrinthitis require urgent surgical intervention to mitigate symptoms and prevent spread to the subarachnoid space or further intracranial complications.

### Intracranial Complications of Otologic Infection

Intracranial complications of mastoiditis are fortunately uncommon in the present era, though it has been suggested that growing antibiotic resistance may play a role in changing incidence.[19] Signs and symptoms may develop in a delayed fashion after an initial course of antibiotics has been administered for otitis media. Symptoms such as headache, nausea, vomiting, diplopia, or nuchal rigidity following otitis media should prompt consideration of imaging to assess for spread of infection beyond the middle ear and mastoid cavity. Use of contrast administration and inclusion of the brain in the scanned field is critical to adequately assess for intracranial involvement.

Otic meningitis may develop through direct spread, hematogenous dissemination, or though thrombosis of dural emissary veins. *Streptococcus pneumoniae* is the leading pathogen in cases of acute otitis media complicated by meningitis. Before widespread vaccination, hemophilus influenzae type B was implicated in most acute cases. *Proteus mirabilis* and *Klebsiella* species are commonly implicated in cases of chronic otitis media or cholesteatoma complicated by meningitis.[20] Diagnosis and bacteriology should be confirmed with lumbar puncture and treatment should consist of culture-directed antibiotic therapy.

Sigmoid sinus thrombosis is an uncommon complication of mastoiditis. In addition to the signs and symptoms associated with mastoiditis, patients may present with worsening headache and cranial neuropathies.[19] Those suspected of having sigmoid sinus thrombosis should undergo imaging, either CT scan with contrast or magnetic resonance angiography (MRA) or magnetic resonance venography (MRV). If unrecognized, venous thrombosis may propagate to the lateral sinus and beyond with significant associated morbidity, including otic hydrocephalus. Underlying infection should be treated surgically. The role of anticoagulation in sigmoid sinus thrombosis remains controversial.[21]

Intracranial abscess is a rare but feared complication of middle ear infection. This may occur as an epidural or subdural abscess. Subdural abscess may be associated with cortical vein thrombosis and result in intracranial hypertension with risk of brainstem herniation. Intracerebral abscess is an extremely rare and morbid complication. Urgent consultation with otolaryngology and neurosurgery is imperative in these settings.

## RHINOLOGIC INFECTIONS

Sinonasal infections have an annual incidence in the United States estimated at 21 million cases, with a cost of greater than $3 billion annually.[22] Almost all upper respiratory infections are viral in nature and self-resolving within 5 to 7 days. Acute bacterial rhinosinusitis (ABRS) typically develops 5 to 7 days after a viral upper respiratory infection with symptoms that include facial pain or pressure, dental pain, retroorbital pain, purulent discharge, and thick postnasal discharge. Fever is uncommon and seen in only about 10% of cases. The triage and management of upper respiratory infections is beyond the scope of this article but is well-described elsewhere.[23,24]

Complications of sinonasal infections are rare but represent clinically urgent or emergent situations that are imperative to diagnose and treat. Spread of infection to the orbital or intracranial spaces is the most common manifestation, whereas systemic spread or sepsis is atypical. Complications of sinonasal infections are thought to occur through thrombophlebitic spread of infection via the epiploic veins that provide communication between the sinuses and orbital and intracranial space.

Although complications are common in children owing to the developing facial skeleton, these infections can also occur in adults. Risk factors include a history of facial trauma with bony fractures, sinus mucocele, immune compromise, diabetes, presence of a skull base defect with or without cerebrospinal fluid leak, and cephalocele.

### Orbital Complications of Acute Sinusitis

Orbital complications of sinusitis are described using the Chandler classification system[25] and include

1. Preseptal cellulitis
2. Orbital cellulitis
3. Subperiosteal orbital abscess (SPOA)
4. Orbital abscess
5. Cavernous sinus thrombosis.

Orbital complications of sinusitis typically develop early in the clinical course and are generally thought not to be preventable.[26]

Preseptal cellulitis presents with edema and erythema of the upper and lower eyelids that accompanies signs and symptoms of acute sinusitis. Soft tissue infection is contained by the orbital septum, a dense fascial aponeurosis that defines the anterior border of the orbit. As an extraorbital process, vision is considered not to be at risk. Rather, the diagnostic imperative is to establish that the orbital contents are not involved. This is accomplished via a thorough ophthalmologic examination, which may be difficult because significant lid edema can render lid retraction challenging. Otolaryngology and ophthalmology consultation is recommended for diagnosis and treatment. Head and neck examination, nasal endoscopy, and ophthalmologic examination may be sufficient for initial diagnosis. Imaging is warranted if there is concern for intraorbital spread or to evaluate the extent of sinus disease. Fine-cut (<1 mm) CT sinus scan is the modality of choice because it provides excellent resolution of sinonasal bony anatomy and soft tissue opacification. Intravenous contrast should be used if there is concern for intraorbital spread of infection.

Treatment of preseptal cellulitis involves intravenous antibiotics (ampicillin-sulbactam [Unasyn] or clindamycin for penicillin allergy; vancomycin may be added for at-risk patients). Inpatient monitoring is warranted and clinical improvement should be noted within 24 to 48 hours, after which an oral antibiotic trial is initiated. Routine eye examination is recommended and clinical deterioration should trigger repeat contrast-enhanced imaging to rule out progression within the orbit.

SPOA is the next most common orbital complication of sinusitis. SPOA occurs with translocation of bacteria through the medial or superior orbital wall via the ethmoid or frontal sinuses, respectively. Signs and symptoms of SPOA include sinonasal and orbital pain, proptosis of the globe, and chemosis of the conjunctiva. Diplopia may occur secondary to displacement of the recti muscles, followed by visual defects, including afferent pupillary or color defects, visual acuity decline, and blindness due to stretch of the optic nerve. Any of these findings should prompt contrast-enhanced CT of the sinuses and orbit. Imaging findings for SPOA include a rim-enhancing fluid collection along the medial or superior orbital wall (**Fig. 4**). Changes to the optic nerve that indicate stretch injury may be seen in more advanced cases.

Treatment of SPOA is based on location, size, and clinical findings. All patients should receive appropriate antibiotics. Small medial SPOA (<6 mm) with minimal (<2 mm) proptosis and no visual impairment may be initially managed with intravenous antibiotics and clinical observation.[27,28] Clinical progression or nonimprovement after 24 to 48 hours of antibiotic therapy should prompt a repeat imaging study. Large (>4–6 mm) medially located SPOAs and superior SPOAs are more likely to fail antibiotic treatment alone and surgical drainage is indicated. Surgical management involves drainage of the SPOA and the sinus of origin.

Orbital cellulitis and cavernous sinus thrombosis constitute ophthalmologic emergencies due to the high rate of blindness and the risk of intracranial spread via the orbital fissures. Significant proptosis and chemosis are typically observed (**Fig. 5**). Visual acuity and pupillary responses are often diminished. Ophthalmoplegia (loss of all extraocular motion) is highly concerning for cavernous sinus involvement. Ophthalmology and otolaryngology consultations should be requested immediately in conjunction with initiation of intravenous antibiotics.

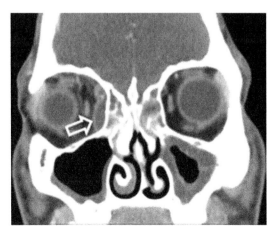

**Fig. 4.** Medial SPOA. Coronal CT scan with contrast demonstrates a medial rim-enhancing fluid collection (*arrow*) with displacement of orbital contents.

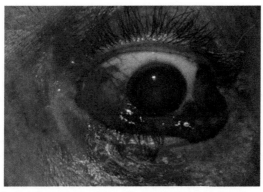

**Fig. 5.** Orbital findings in a patient with orbital cellulitis and cavernous sinus thrombosis. Note the proptosis and chemosis. This patient also has ophthalmoplegia.

### Intracranial Complications of Acute Sinusitis

Intracranial complications of ABRS include meningitis, epidural abscess, subdural abscess, cerebritis, and cerebral abscess. Additional risk factors for these complications include a history of head or facial trauma, immune compromise, presence of a skull base defect, and cephalocele. Although a comprehensive discussion of the management and workup of intracranial infections is beyond the scope of this article, health care providers should be cognizant of the possibility of sinonasal source in patients with these conditions. Patients with concern for intracranial infection should be evaluated and treated with current best practice standards.

Patients with meningeal signs, seizures, motor or sensory deficits, or nonresolving severe headaches in conjunction with ABRS should undergo a fine-cut CT with contrast and MRI with gadolinium of the face or sinuses. A CT sinus scan allows for the evaluation of subtle bony defects of the cribriform plate, ethmoid roof, and sphenoid sinus. Use of contrast allows for assessment of rim-enhancing fluid collections. MRI is advantageous for distinguishing between fluid within a sinus and cephalocele, which is critical to identify before surgical intervention.

### Invasive Fungal Sinusitis

Invasive fungal sinusitis is a rare but devastating disease. The infectious agent is typically *Aspergillus* or *Mucorales* species, both of which are ubiquitous in nature, and generally account for chronic and acute fulminant infections, respectively. Relative or absolute neutropenia is the principle risk factor for invasive infection.[29] Diabetic ketoacidosis, myeloablative chemotherapy, prolonged high-dose steroid use, or posttransplant immunosuppression are frequently present and a high-index of suspicion should be maintained with these patient populations.

Acute fulminant invasive fungal sinusitis (AFIFS) should be distinguished from noninvasive fungal infections. Mycetomas are inspissated collections of mucoid and fungal debris that become entrapped within a sinus and have the characteristic imaging findings of calcifications in the obstructed sinus on CT scan or T1-weighted or T2-weighted hypointensity on MRI. Allergic fungal sinusitis is a separate and distinct entity that exhibits hypereosinophilic reaction and nasal polyp formation in response to fungal colonization. These 2 entities should not be confused with AFIFS because the prognosis of noninvasive disease is favorable.

The pathophysiology underlying precipitation of fungal invasion remains controversial. Violation of the mucocutaneous barrier in a neutropenic patient is a clear risk factor for initiation of these infections; acute bacterial sinusitis, dental work, and trauma are also known to be precipitating factors. In the absence of neutrophilic defenses, entry of *Rhizopus* or *Mucorales* species through the mucocutaneous barrier precipitates an acute, fulminant angioinvasive infection that extends via vascular networks. Progression of infection is exceedingly fast. Initial symptoms may mimic acute bacterial sinusitis, including facial pain and pressure; congestion; headache; and fever. However, within days, invasion of nearby structures, including the orbit and intracranium, along with cranial nerves, may result in facial paresthesia, diplopia, proptosis, chemosis, ophthalmoplegia, and vision loss.

Mortality rates for AFIFS range from 20% to 80%, with a 100% fatality rate if left untreated.[30] Extent of spread, reversibility of immune dysfunction, and tolerance of antifungal medications are the primary factors affecting survivability. For example, a delay in diagnosis of greater than 5 days is an independent risk factor for mortality in AFIFS, with 80% of those patients succumbing to the disease.[31] Intracranial involvement and advanced age have also been shown to be independent poor prognosticators for survival.[32]

As such, early recognition and treatment is critical to improving outcomes in AFIFS, and a high index of suspicion is required to make the diagnosis. Head and neck examination, nasal endoscopy, and MRI with gadolinium are the gold standard. Neutropenic patients with new-onset sinonasal symptoms or fever of unknown origin and CT scan findings suggestive of sinusitis should undergo urgent MRI of the face or sinus with gadolinium. Loss of contrast enhancement (LoCE) is the hallmark radiologic feature of invasive fungal infections on MRI.[33] LoCE is characterized by a region of sinonasal mucosa, which normally shows enhancement on T1-weighted postgadolinium-MRI sequences but instead appears dark with extensive surrounding inflammatory changes (**Fig. 6**).

Successful treatment of invasive fungal sinusitis relies on 3 pillars: antifungal medication, surgical debridement of necrotic tissues, and reversal of neutropenic deficit. Immediate initiation of liposomal amphotericin B can slow the rapid progression of

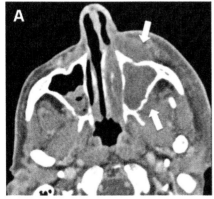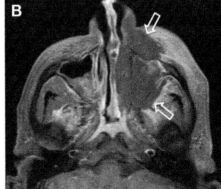

**Fig. 6.** Imaging findings in invasive fungal sinusitis. (*A*) An axial CT scan with contrast demonstrating sinus opacification and fat stranding in the premalar and retromaxillary spaces (*solid arrows*). (*B*) An axial postgadolinium T1-weighted MRI demonstrating LoCE with central hypointensity, indicating a region of necrosis (*open arrows*).

angioinvasion and allow time for transfer to higher level of care, surgical planning, and goals of care discussion.

## SUMMARY

Infections of the head and neck are common and, in most cases, may be appropriately managed by the primary care provider. However, one should be aware of the presenting features of complicated head and neck infections; in many cases, timely recognition is critical to prevent significant morbidity. Concern for development of a complicated or aggressive infection should prompt urgent otolaryngology consultation. Initiation of medical management and evaluation with appropriate imaging are important first steps in facilitating care. Transfer of care to tertiary level facilities should be considered to facilitate multidisciplinary treatment where services are otherwise unavailable.

## REFERENCES

1. CDC Summary health statistics: national health interview survey, 2016. Available at: https://ftp.cdc.gov/pub/Health_Statistics/NCHS/NHIS/SHS/2016_SHS_Table_A-2.pdf. Accessed June 18, 2018.
2. Taylor S, Marchisio P, Vergison A, et al. Impact of pneumococcal conjugate vaccination on otitis media: a systematic review. Clin Infect Dis 2012;54(12):1765–73.
3. National Center for Health Statistics. National ambulatory medical care survey: 1998 summary. 2000. Available at: http://www.cdc.gov/nchs/. Accessed August 1, 2016.
4. Hidaka H, Yamaguchi T, Hasegawa J, et al. Clinical and bacteriological influence of diabetes mellitus on deep neck infection: systematic review and meta-analysis. Head Neck 2015;37:1536–46.
5. Cramer JD, Purkey MR, Smith SS, et al. The impact of delayed surgical drainage of deep neck abscesses in adult and pediatric populations. Laryngoscope 2016; 126:1753–60.
6. Boscolo-Rizzo P, Stetlin M, Muzzi E, et al. Deep neck infections: a study of 365 cases highlighting recommendations for management and treatment. Eur Arch Otorhinolaryngol 2012;269(4):1241–9.
7. Freeman RK, Vallières E, Verrier ED, et al. Descending necrotizing mediastinitis: an analysis of the effects of serial surgical debridement on patient mortality. J Thorac Cardiovasc Surg 2000;119(2):260–7.
8. Martins JR, Chagas OL Jr, Velasques BD, et al. The use of antibiotics in odontogenic infections: what is the best choice? a systematic review. J Oral Maxillofac Surg 2017;75(12):2606.e1-11.
9. Johnson R, Stewart M. The contemporary approach to diagnosis and management of peritonsillar abscess. Curr Opin Otolaryngol Head Neck Surg 2005; 13(3):157–60.
10. Ito K, Chitose H, Koganemaru M. Four cases of acute epiglottitis with a peritonsillar abscess. Auris Nasus Larynx 2011;38(2):284–8.
11. Schubert AD, Hotz MA, Caversaccio MD, et al. Septic thrombosis of the internal jugular vein: Lemierre's syndrome revisited. Laryngoscope 2015;125(4):863–8.
12. Thakur JS, Verma N, Thakur A, et al. Necrotizing cervical fasciitis: prognosis based on a new grading system. Ear Nose Throat J 2013;92(3):149–52.
13. Klabacha ME, Stankiewicz JA, Clift SE. Severe soft tissue infection of the face and neck: a classification. Laryngoscope 1982;92(10 Pt 1):1135–9.
14. Panda NK, Simhadri S, Sridhara SR. Cervicofacial necrotizing fasciitis: can we expect a favourable outcome? J Laryngol Otol 2004;118(10):771–7.

15. Gliklich RE, Eavey RD, Iannuzzi RA, et al. A contemporary analysis of acute mastoiditis. Arch Otolaryngol Head Neck Surg 1996;122(2):135–9.
16. Pang LHY, Barakate MS, Havas TE. Mastoiditis in a paediatric population: a review of 11 years experience in management. Int J Pediatr Otorhinolaryngol 2009;73(11):1520–4.
17. Ghadersohi S, Young NM, Smith-Bronstein V, et al. Management of acute complicated mastoiditis at an urban, tertiary care pediatric hospital. Laryngoscope 2017;127(10):2321–7.
18. Spiegel JH, Lustig LR, Lee KC, et al. Contemporary presentation and management of a spectrum of mastoid abscesses. Laryngoscope 1998;108(6):822–8.
19. Osborn AJ, Blaser S, Papsin BC. Decisions regarding intracranial complications from acute mastoiditis in children. Curr Opin Otolaryngol Head Neck Surg 2011; 19(6):478–85.
20. Slovik Y, Kraus M, Leiberman A, et al. Role of surgery in the management of otogenic meningitis. J Laryngol Otol 2007;121(9):897–901.
21. Mather M, Musgrave K, Dawe N. Is anticoagulation beneficial in acute mastoiditis complicated by sigmoid sinus thrombosis? Laryngoscope 2018. https://doi.org/10.1002/lary.27151.
22. Marple BF, Brunton S, Ferguson BJ. Acute bacterial rhinosinusitis: a review of U.S. treatment guidelines. Otolaryngol Head Neck Surg 2006;135(3):341–8.
23. Chow AW, Benninger MS, Brook I, et al. IDSA clinical practice guideline for acute bacterial rhinosinusitis in children and adults. Clin Infect Dis 2012;54(8):e72–112.
24. Rosenfeld RM, Piccirillo JF, Chandrasekhar SS, et al. Clinical practice guideline (update): adult sinusitis. Otolaryngol Head Neck Surg 2015;152(4):598–609.
25. Chandler JR, Langenbrunner DJ, Stevens ER. The pathogenesis of orbital complications in acute sinusitis. Laryngoscope 1970;80:1418–20.
26. Sinclair CF, Berkowitz RG. Prior antibiotic therapy for acute sinusitis in children and the development of subperiosteal orbital abscess. Int J Pediatr Otorhinolaryngol 2007;71(7):1003–6.
27. Rahbar R, Robson CD, Petersen RA, et al. Management of orbital subperiosteal abscess in children. Arch Otolaryngol Head Neck Surg 2001;127(3):281–6.
28. Oxford LE, McClay J. Medical and surgical management of subperiosteal orbital abscess secondary to acute sinusitis in children. Int J Pediatr Otorhinolaryngol 2006;70(11):1853–61.
29. Petrikkos G, Skiada A, Lortholary O, et al. Epidemiology and clinical manifestations of mucormycosis. Clin Infect Dis 2012;54(Suppl 1):S23–34.
30. Gillespie MB, O'Malley BW Jr, Francis HW. An approach to fulminant invasive fungal rhinosinusitis in the immunocompromised host. Arch Otolaryngol Head Neck Surg 1998;124(5):520–6.
31. Walsh TJ, Gamaletsou MN, McGinnis MR, et al. Early clinical and laboratory diagnosis of invasive pulmonary, extrapulmonary, and disseminated mucormycosis (zygomycosis). Clin Infect Dis 2012;54(Suppl 1):S55–60.
32. Turner JH, Soudry E, Nayak JV, et al. Survival outcomes in acute invasive fungal sinusitis: a systematic review and quantitative synthesis of published evidence. Laryngoscope 2013;123(5):1112–8.
33. Groppo ER, El-Sayed IH, Aiken AH, et al. Computed tomography and magnetic resonance imaging characteristics of acute invasive fungal sinusitis. Arch Otolaryngol Head Neck Surg 2011;137(10):1005–10.

# Speech Language Pathology Rehabilitation

Kristine Pietsch, MA, CCC-SLP[a], Tiffany Lyon, MS, CCC-SLP[b], Vaninder K. Dhillon, MD[a,c],*

## KEYWORDS

- Speech language pathology • Dysphonia • Dysphagia • Stroke • Fluency

## KEY POINTS

- The speech language pathologist (SLP) has a vital management role in patients with voice and swallow concerns, as well as stroke patients and patients with fluency problems.
- An SLP has a multiplicity of roles, and this article summarizes the variety of speech and swallow rehabilitation that adult patients may require or seek if they are under the treatment of an SLP.
- The case examples allow the reader to base the clinical decision-making process within the context of a patient presentation and elucidate the role of speech and language pathology services for the primary care provider in order to refer patients with symptoms and concerns to the right provider early in their medical care.

## REHABILITATION IN PATIENTS WITH DYSPHONIA

Case example: 32-year-old woman who presented with 3-month history of persistent dysphonia. She worked as a bartender at a local concert venue part-time while taking musical theater classes on the side. She started her musical theater classes approximately 5 months previous, which required her to sing at least 10 to 15 hours a week. As a bartender, she worked most weekends over loud noise. She noticed a raspy quality to her voice with voice breaks, and over the previous 2 months, difficulty in reaching her high range. After a weekend of working she reported losing her voice and a longer recovery time during the week, affecting her musical theater classes. She reported some odynophonia during the weekends. No swallow or breathing complaints. She did not report smoking.

Conflict of Interest: None of the authors of this article have any commercial or financial conflicts of interest to disclose. None of the authors have any funding sources that contribute to the publication of this article.

[a] Department of Otolaryngology, Johns Hopkins University, 601 North Caroline Street, 6th Floor, Baltimore, MD 21287, USA; [b] Department of Speech and Language Pathology, University of Utah, 50 North Medical Drive, Salt Lake City, UT 84132, USA; [c] Department of Otolaryngology Head and Neck Surgery, Johns Hopkins University, National Capital Region, 6420 Rockledge Drive, Suite 4920, Bethesda, MD 20817, USA

* Corresponding author. Department of Otolaryngology Head and Neck Surgery, Johns Hopkins University, National Capital Region, 6420 Rockledge Drive, Suite 4920, Bethesda, MD 20817.

E-mail address: Vdhillo2@jhmi.edu

## Introduction

The burden of dysphonia rests on primary care clinics. Most patients (90%) initially present to primary care physicians with dysphonia.[1,2] Primary care providers can elicit important initial questions in the history in order to guide the timing for referral to the speech language pathologist (SLP).

### What is the duration of the dysphonia?

According to the 2018 revised guidelines on dysphonia per the American Academy of Otolaryngology Head and Neck Surgery (AAOHNS) there is a recommendation for referral to laryngologist for fiberoptic evaluation if dysphonia persists beyond 4 weeks duration.[3] According to the American Academy of Family Physicians (AAFP), published recommendations indicate referral to an otolaryngologist between 2 weeks and 3 months of dysphonia.[4] It is important that any patient with persistent dysphonia, and those who are voice professionals or heavy voice users, are referred to laryngologists as well as SLPs for direct visualization of the larynx.

For self-limiting causes of dysphonia, more commonly acute laryngitis, the resolution of voice symptoms should occur within 1 to 3 weeks.[5] The most common cause of laryngitis is viral, and therefore there is no recommendation for antibiotics or steroids. Symptomatic relief and time should cause resolution.

### Does the dysphonia cause communication problems?

Professional voice users, including teachers, singers and lecturers should be evaluated for voice concerns in relationship to their communication needs. Singers are expectedly more anxious about their voice problems,[6,7] and seek early consultation for dysphonia. For those whose voice is affecting their occupation, early referral to a specialist is advised.

### Are there associated symptoms including dysphagia, breathing complaints, hemoptysis, otalgia and/or stridor, or recent surgical procedure of the head or neck, or any procedure with intubation?

Patients with associated symptoms listed should trigger early referral for specialty evaluation with fiberoptic laryngoscopy. The complication frequency to the recurrent laryngeal nerve is high in patients who undergo thyroidectomy and cervical spine surgery.[8,9] Patients presenting with new-onset postoperative dysphonia should have an expedited laryngeal evaluation, which is recommended between 2 weeks and 2 months of surgery, according to the AAOHNS.[10] A systematic review demonstrated that intubation can cause clinically relevant complications related to short-term general anesthesia with tube or laryngeal mask, and therefore concern for laryngeal injury after intubation should be investigated.[11]

## Evaluation

The AAOHNS dysphonia guidelines give a strong recommendation for direct visualization of the larynx over any other modality of work up.[3] The importance of an appropriate diagnosis ensures adequate and appropriate treatment. The role of stroboscopy (endoscopy with stroboscopy that allows for vocal fold wave motion analysis) in particular has been shown to change the diagnosis of dysphonia in up to 56% of cases,[1] thereby changing the course of management.[12–14]

## Treatment

Based upon observational studies, small-sample randomized control studies, and expert opinion (and high confidence) the AAOHNS recommends vocal hygiene play an important part of any treatment plan.[3] Vocal hygiene includes hydration, humidification, improving aggravating factors, and irritants that may cause vocal abuse/misuse or laryngeal hypersensitivity.

Voice therapy is widely accepted as the first line and most conservative form of treatment for benign etiologies of dysphonia. When voice therapy cannot improve subjective voice-related quality of life and/or objective vocal parameters in patients with phonotraumatic lesions, then surgery is recommended.[15]

Voice therapy includes direct and indirect approaches. Indirect therapy encompasses hygiene recommendations, and/or counseling regarding compensation or use of amplification devices. Direct approaches aim to alter physiology to restore improved quality and/or function and facilitate healing of mucosa through exercise.[16–18] Direct approaches will include changes in posture, respiratory control, phonation, articulation, resonance, and muscle tension through various techniques.

---

The patient was referred to a laryngologist who completed a stroboscopy, which showed evidence of a vocal fold polyp. Given the size of the polyp, she was referred to speech language pathology. Compensatory strategies and vocal hygiene were implemented as part of her voice therapy, and over the course of 1 to 2 months, her voice started to improve. She also quit her job as a bartender and started working in retail. On follow-up with her primary care physician, she stated her voice improved, and her polyp was resolving. She reported that she planned to continue with voice therapy for another month as recommended by the therapist and laryngologist. She was happy with the improvement in her voice and with the guidance she received from the SLP and laryngologist.

---

### Conclusion

In conclusion, dysphonia is a common and prevalent symptom that is seen in primary care clinics. The role of speech therapy in dysphonia is a routine adjunct whether or not surgical management is indicative. Guidelines on voice therapy, including voice rest postoperatively, are evolving, but in patients seen for dysphonia, a referral for voice therapy is the recommended standard of conservative management.

### REHABILITATION IN PATIENTS WITH DYSPHAGIA

---

Case example: an 85-year-old woman with PMH of mild hypertension and chronic obstructive pulmonary disease (COPD) presented for a wellness check following a recent hospitalization. She sustained a hip fracture 6 months ago, and since that time has been wheelchair bound. A respiratory illness resulted in her most recent hospitalization, where she was diagnosed with pneumonia and treated with antibiotics. Chest radiograph revealed infiltrate in the right lower lobe, suggestive of aspiration. She reported coughing on thin liquids over the past several months, multiple times per day. She used to be able to take several pills at once, but now has more difficulty and has been taking them one at a time and cutting some larger pills in half.

---

### Introduction

Dysphagia is the symptom of difficulty or discomfort while swallowing. Swallowing is a complex act, categorized into 3 phases: oral preparatory phase, pharyngeal phase, and esophageal phase. Underlying etiologic factors for oropharyngeal dysphagia include any disease processes that negatively impacts cranial nerves V, VII, IX, X, XI, XII, or otherwise change the anatomy and physiology of the structures of the face, mouth, velum, pharynx, larynx, or upper esophageal sphincter.[19,20]

Oropharyngeal swallowing dysfunction is estimated to impact 16 million Americans, and the negative consequences of insufficient treatment can result in dehydration, starvation, aspiration pneumonia, and airway obstruction.[21] Aspiration pneumonia is a primary cause of mortality in patients with neurogenic dysphagia, and accounts for 13% to 48% of all infections in nursing home residents.[22] Silent aspiration, defined as aspiration of food, liquid, or saliva that does not generate an airway protection response from the patient, is a common finding in individuals with a history of head and neck cancer, neurologic impairment, and gastrointestinal disease and may not generate dysphagia complaints.[23] In this case, a diagnosis of aspiration pneumonia, dehydration, or unexplained weight loss may serve as r primary referral triggers.

### Evaluation

The diagnosis of oropharyngeal dysphagia calls for a multidisciplinary approach, and will often include not only SLP and otolaryngologists, but gastroenterologists, neurologists, geriatric internists, and radiologists. An SLP evaluation of dysphagia begins with a comprehensive medical and symptom history, as well as observations of patient's ability to follow directions and mental status.[22,24] The SLP then chooses the method of evaluating swallow function dependent upon several factors. There are a series of common measures and rating scales used clinically and in outcomes research that can be used for objective assessment of swallow (**Table 1**).[25] Visualization of the swallow can be obtained endoscopically (fiberoptic endoscopic evaluation of swallowing - FEES) or via videofluoroscopy (modified barium swallow study - MBS). The SLP will determine which manner of evaluation is most appropriate for the patient in order to make treatment recommendations (**Table 2**).

### Treatment

SLP treatment approaches for dysphagia will include some combination of diet recommendations, exercises designed to improve strength, range of motion and coordination of the swallowing mechanism, compensatory maneuvers, and

| Table 1 | |
|---|---|
| **Common measures and rating scales used clinically and in outcomes research** | |
| Penetration Aspiration Scale (PAS) (Rosenbek, Robbins, Roecker, Coyle, & Wood, 1996) | An 8-point, equal appearing interval scale to describe penetration and aspiration events. 1- no penetration or aspiration to 8- silent aspiration |
| Functional Oral Intake Scale (FOIS) (M. A. Crary, Carnaby Mann, & Groher, 2005) | 7-point ordinal scale scale to document change in functional oral intake of food and liquid. 1- nothing by mouth to 7- total oral diet with no restrictions |
| Modified Barium Swallow Impairment Profile (MBSimp) (Martin-Harris et al., 2008) | Quantifies visual observations of swallowing impairment during the MBSS with a scoring system of 17 components with numeric correlates for distinct physiologic observations |
| Iowa Oral Performance Instrument (Adams, Mathisen, Baines, Lazarus, & Callister, 2015) | Allows for quantitative assessment for tongue and lip strength in kPa with normative values |

**Table 2**
Evaluation techniques for oropharyngeal swallow

| Evaluation Name | Procedures | Pros | Cons | Who Is It Best for? |
|---|---|---|---|---|
| Clinical/Bedside Swallow Examination | • Patient takes food, liquid of different consistencies<br>• 3 ounce water swallow protocol<br>• Compensatory maneuvers may be implemented facilitate symptom improvement | • Low cost<br>• Non invasive<br>• Natural environment; observing swallowing in the context of a meal<br>• No radiation | • No observation of physiology<br>• Cannot rule out silent aspiration | Patients who:<br>• Are likely to have good sensation<br>• Cannot be moved<br>• Cannot receive radiation and/or cannot tolerate endoscopy |
| Fiberoptic Endoscopic Evaluation of Swallowing | Patient takes food, liquid of different consistencies while undergoing endoscopy<br>• Compensatory maneuvers may be implemented | • Does not require pt transport/can be done at bedside<br>• Real food<br>• Can assess pharyngeal physiology, including vocal fold motion/closure<br>• Can assess aspiration/penetration before and after the swallow, can assess residue in pharynx<br>• Can appreciate differences in anatomy following surgery, XRT<br>• Can choose to assess sensation | • Can't evaluate oral phase.<br>• Cannot assess aspiration *during* the swallow or UES opening due to "white out" at the moment of swallow<br>• Patient discomfort | Patients who:<br>• Demonstrate overt s/s of dysphagia on clinical swallow, more information needed<br>• Have known or suspected sensory deficits<br>• Have altered anatomy following surgery<br>• Could benefit from biofeedback to learn compensatory strategies<br>• Impaired sensation/history of silent aspiration |

*(continued on next page)*

**Table 2**
*(continued)*

| Evaluation Name | Procedures | Pros | Cons | Who Is It Best for? |
|---|---|---|---|---|
| Modified Barium Swallow/ Videofluoroscopic Swallowing Study | • Patient takes barium infused food, liquid of different consistencies while seated or standing in lateral, anteroposterior and sometimes oblique positions<br>• Compensatory maneuvers may be implemented<br>• Done in conjunction with a radiologist | • Oral, pharyngeal and some esophageal physiology and timing measures can be assessed throughout the entirety of the swallow<br>• Can assess aspiration/ penetration during all parts of the swallow<br>• Can infer sensation with cough responsiveness<br>• Can assess cricopharyngeal function<br>• In some settings, can screen esophageal phase | • Cannot assess vocal fold motion/closure<br>• Cannot directly assess sensation<br>• Not available at all facilities<br>• Requires transport<br>• Radiation exposure<br>• Barium taste | Patients who:<br>• Have suspected oral phase or pharyngoesophageal deficits<br>• Cannot tolerate endoscopy<br>• Have impaired sensation/ history of silent aspiration<br>• May benefit from exercises/maneuvers |

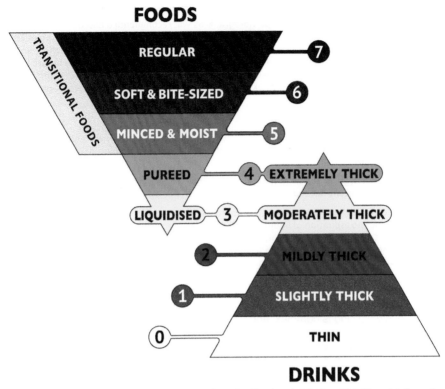

**Fig. 1.** The International Dysphagia Diet Standardisation initiative (IDDSI) guidelines for food and liquid consistencies. (*From* The international dysphagia diet standardisation initiative 2016.

behavioral or lifestyle changes. The SLP should provide guidance for food and liquid consistencies judged to be most appropriate for the patient based on the results of the swallowing evaluation. New guidelines for food and liquid consistencies have recently been recommended by the International Dysphagia Diet Standardisation initiative (IDDSI), with the intent of making it easier for patients, families, and other care providers to judge whether food or liquid items adhere to the prescribed diet[26] (**Fig. 1**).

### Compensatory Techniques and Swallowing Exercises

Postural techniques (eg, chin tuck, head tilt, or head turn to 1 side) aimed at improving airway protection or facilitating bolus transit are commonly recommended as temporary or longer-term strategies to attenuate the effects of dysphagia.[27] Swallowing exercises are employed to address particular muscle groups and physiologic outcomes, ranging from increases in pharyngeal constriction, base of tongue retraction, elevation and anterior movement of the hyolaryngeal complex, and UES opening. Most swallowing program recommendations follow general exercise physiology and motor learning principles, recommending at minimum daily home practice of multiple sets of exercises, with 5 to 6 weeks of once- to twice-weekly sessions for outpatient services.[28,29]

The patient was referred to a speech pathologist. MBS was recommended based on a desire to further evaluate physiology for treatment planning. MBS revealed loss of part of the bolus to the pharynx before initiation of the pharyngeal swallow, weak base of tongue retraction, and pharyngeal constriction resulting in penetration and trace aspiration of thin liquids before the swallow. Penetration aspiration scale score (PAS) was 7. Use of a chin tuck maneuver eliminated aspiration. The patient received a 5-week course of swallowing therapy, during which time she was counseled to

1. Use a chin tuck for all thin or nectar thick liquids

2. Engage in daily exercise using Masako maneuver and effortful swallow to target base of tongue retraction and pharyngeal constriction, as well as EMST training to improve cough strength

3. Optimize oral hygiene and work with physical therapy to optimize her cardiovascular health in light of her recent deconditioning

A repeat MBS following therapy resulted in improvements in swallowing physiology, with flash penetration but no aspiration of liquids (PAS 2). Functionally, she no longer exhibited coughing with liquids. Chin tuck use was discontinued, with recommendations to continue physical exercise and oral hygiene, and to return if she noted any return of symptoms of dysphagia.

## Conclusion

The act of swallowing is complex, and optimal function of all phases of the swallow is crucial in the ability to receive adequate nutrition and hydration and protect the airway. Dysphagia can negatively impact overall health and quality of life. Adequate assessment and personalized, evidence-based treatment by a swallowing team, including the SLP and otolaryngologist, are crucial to facilitating good outcomes in this population.

## REHABILITATION AFTER STROKE

Case study: a 55-year-old gentleman with a history of hypertension, smoking, and 2 previous transient ischemic attacks (TIA) who had a stroke. On admission to the emergency room, the patient had sudden-onset dysphonia and was screened, resulting in an ear, nose, and throat (ENT) consult. ENT saw patient on day 1 after admission and diagnosed the patient with a left vocal fold, lingual, pharyngeal, and palatal paralysis severely impairing the patient's ability to swallow and speak. He was placed on diet restrictions with nothing by mouth (NPO), and SLP evaluation was ordered. Because of difficulty ambulating, a FEES was performed at bedside and documented silent aspiration on all consistencies. The patient had a gastric tube placed, and enteral feeds were recommended primarily for nutrition. The patient was discharged to an acute care rehabilitation center and scheduled to follow-up with his primary care provider within 48 hours of inpatient discharge.

## Introduction

The primary care physician plays a crucial role in coordinating care across specialties after the patient has been discharged from the inpatient hospital. The 2018 Guidelines for Management of Acute Ischemic Stroke published by the American Heart Association (AHA) and the American Stroke Association (ASA) strongly recommend that all stroke patients receive "formal assessment of their activities of daily living and instrumental activities of daily living, communication abilities, and functional mobility before discharge from acute care hospitalization and the findings be incorporated into the care transition and the discharge planning process."[30] An evaluation with a qualified SLP is necessary to determine if therapy services are warranted, what deficits can be remediated, how long the patient might anticipate for recovery, and/or what impairments by be long lasting and require compensatory management.

### Evaluation

The primary care physician's assessment of a stroke patient upon discharge from the hospital requires a conversation with the patient and family about the patient's goals and setting reasonable expectations about functional improvements. A cranial nerve examination to screen for weakness or discoordination of the palate, tongue, and lips can direct the physician's attention to issues that may need further assessment and management by an ENT, specialty voice and swallowing center, or prosthodontist. It is important that every stroke patient with deficits in swallow, voice, or with evidence of cranial neuropathy be evaluated by an otolaryngologist.

### Treatment

A therapy plan is then developed based on the analysis of testing and joint goal-setting with the patient and caregivers. For patients whose symptoms do not resolve in the first 2 weeks, it can take between 2 to 3 months to show signs of improvement,[31] and some patients who do not display signs of swallow impairment at 3 months can present again at 6 months with difficulties swallowing. Swallowing should be closely monitored and evaluated throughout the recovery process. If the voice is altered, this should also be closely monitored and if there is no recovery, patients should be referred to an otolaryngologist for direct visualization.

Cognitive impairments following a stroke can occur in about 20% to 30% of patients at 3 months after stroke, and were unchanged at 12 months follow-up according to Douiri, and colleagues.[32] SLP therapy techniques have been developed to manage and compensate for various cognitive impairments, including memory, executive functioning, problem solving, and attention. A review of 370 studies between the years of 2003 and 2008 concluded that cognitive exercises and strategies can be beneficial for patients with mild-to-severe impairments, but the type of interventions should vary based on severity.[33]

---

The patient was evaluated by an SLP in the acute care rehabilitation center who noted anomia, ataxic dysarthria, and apraxia of speech in addition to dysphagia. Over the course of 3 weeks of intensive daily therapy, the patient was able to progress to tolerating a puree diet, nectar thick liquids, and free thin water while adhering to an oral hygiene protocol every 4 to 6 hours. The patient was referred to an outpatient laryngology clinic for management of left vocal fold paralysis who offered a vocal fold bulking injection, which was expected to last 3 to 6 months. Although still PEG dependent for nutrition, it is expected that the patient will regain the ability to swallow by mouth within the next 3 to 4 months by using a combination of compensatory strategies and strengthening exercises. The speech therapist has designed a treatment plan including progressive lingual-strengthening exercises, swallowing exercises, word retrieval strategies, and speech exercises to improve coordination and clarity of speech. Therapy will continue twice weekly for 6 to 8 weeks.

---

### Conclusion

Primary care physicians can improve the quality and management of their poststroke patients' cognitive, communicative, and swallowing function by appropriately screening and referring for the impairments discussed in this article. Only an evaluation with a competent and specialized speech pathologist will determine the extent to which patients will require and benefit from speech pathology services. Establishing strong relationships with the SLPs in the community will allow understanding of their areas of expertise, and facilitate the best possible care for patients.

## REHABILITATION FOR FLUENCY

A 45-year-old man presented to clinic with new onset of stuttering. It began following the sudden death of a family member. Although already engaged in grief counseling to address the loss, his fluency did not improve after several weeks of therapy. He worked as a call center operator, and the frequent repetitions and hesitations in his speech made it difficult to communicate with customers.

### Introduction

Disfluencies are present in the everyday speech of all normal individuals, occurring on approximately 1% of uttered syllables.[34,35] These disfluencies can form meaningless words, phrases, or sounds that mark a pause or hesitation in speech, such as "uh" or "um". To be labeled with a fluency disorder, an individual can demonstrate excessive numbers of these types of fillers in conversation, but will also present with more atypical disfluencies, such as

1. Sound (m-m-m-mom), syllable (fa-fa-fa-father) or whole word repetitions (boy-boy-boy)
2. Prolongations of a single sound (mmmmmmy)
3. Blocks where a period of tense silence with frozen articulatory posture is demonstrated before initiating sound ([lips placed together]………….my)
4. Broken words, with inappropriate pause between syllables (o-pen)

Diagnosis of a fluency disorder is made when more than 3% of syllables are stuttered.[34] Secondary behaviors such as facial grimacing, eye blinking, or other motor tics during stuttering events are common in people who stutter.[35]

Stuttering severity will vary widely within an individual, and can be influenced by situations, settings, conversational partners, lexical complexity, and-most notably-anxiety. It is common for people who stutter to complain of an increase of stuttering events when faced with speaking on the phone, saying their own name, or when presented with particular speech sounds.

Fluency disorders are broadly categorized as developmental stuttering or acquired stuttering. Acquired stuttering presents later than developmental stuttering, most commonly secondary to neurologic event such as stroke or traumatic brain injury, with a smaller percentage being psychogenic in origin. Acquired stuttering can arise from damage to nearly any part of the brain,[36] and most who develop fluency issues as a result of neurologic event also had concomitant speech disorders such as aphasia, dysarthria, or apraxia of speech. Reports of acquired fluency disorders attributed to medication side effect found fluency returned after the medication was discontinued.[37] An estimated half of neurogenic stutterers resolve without intervention.[38] Etiology of stuttering can be most reliably identified by onset of symptoms, although it is important to note developmental stuttering can re-emerge in adulthood in the absence of symptoms for years, often because of new stressors.[39]

### Treatment

Treatment recommendations for adults who stutter fall into 3 primary categories: fluency enhancing,[40,41] stuttering modification,[42] and anxiety reduction or emotional resilience approaches. The general consensus is supportive of a blended approach that uses history, current presentation of symptoms, and the patient's goals to develop a treatment plan and provide individualized care. Large randomized double-blind studies of various treatment paradigms are absent from the fluency literature.

### Treatment Length and Intensity

Stuttering therapy is often administered in the context of intensive multiweek programs with individual as well as group sessions, but can also follow a more traditional therapy schedule of 1 to 2 sessions per week for several months.[43] Patients who stuttermay go through several courses of speech intervention in their lifetime. There are several well-documented fluency-enhancing conditions, including: speaking when alone, speaking with a reduced rate, speaking in time to a rhythmic stimulus, choral reading, singing, speaking in a novel pattern, reading, and speaking under altered auditory feedback.[44] Patients should choose approaches that fit their particular goals at the time of seeking treatment, and consider involvement in support groups such as the National Stuttering Association for lifelong support and updates in evidence-based treatment options.[45]

---

The patient underwent outpatient evaluation, where he received an overall score of 26 on the SSI-4, consistent with moderate stuttering. His overall impact OASES score was 3.09, indicating that his stuttering was having a moderate-to-severe impact on his quality of life. A discussion of the patient's history was positive for stuttering as a child, which resolved spontaneously without intervention. The patient and the speech pathologist discussed his test results and stated goals for communication, which were solely to improve fluency on the phone at work. They ultimately decided on an intensive fluency-enhancing approach of 3 1 hour sessions per week. After 2 weeks, the patient was feeling confident in his ability to implement fluency-enhancing techniques of light articulatory contacts, reduced rate, and optimized breath support and was able to successfully implement these techniques in his job duties. As he continued to implement strategies and concurrently receive counseling services for his recent traumatic life event, he experienced a complete resolution of symptoms.

---

### Conclusion

Stuttering is a complex neurologic phenomenon, and understanding of its etiology continues to develop. Most stuttering is developmental in nature. If stuttering emerges in adulthood, it is likely secondary to a neurologic event, relapse/exacerbation of childhood stuttering, psychiatric in nature, or a medication side effect. A patient may have multiple courses of stuttering therapy to manage relapsing and remitting symptoms across the lifespan. Group therapy is common, and support groups such as the National Stuttering Association can offer support and advocacy for individuals with chronic fluency disorders.

### SUMMARY

In conclusion, rehabilitation with speech and language pathology can take many forms. The role of speech and language pathology is crucial in the management of patients with dysphonia and dysphagia, even if the primary modality of treatment may be surgical or medical management. Multiple treatment guidelines illustrate the importance and strong recommendation for speech and language pathology in addressing the needs of patients with voice and swallow concerns, as well as in the rehabilitation of poststroke patients and those with fluency disorders. It is important to keep in mind that referral patterns should remain robust and fluid between primary care, otolaryngologists, and other providers with the speech and language pathology community, so that patients are not delayed in receiving rehabilitation.

## REFERENCES

1. Cohen SM, Kim J, Roy N, et al. Factors influencing referral of patients with voice disorders from primary care to otolaryngology. Laryngoscopy 2014;124:21–220.
2. Cohen SM, Kim J, Roy N, et al. Delayed otolaryngology referral for voice disorders increases health care costs. Am J Med 2015;128:426.e11-8.
3. Stachler RJ, Francis DO, Schwartz SR, et al. Clinical practice guideline: hoarseness (Dysphonia) update. Otolaryngol Head Neck Surg 2018;158(1_suppl):S1–42.
4. House SA, Fisher EL. Hoarseness in adults. Am Fam Physician 2017;96(11):720–8.
5. Dworkin JP. Laryngitis: types, causes and treatments. Otolaryngol Clin North Am 2008;41:419–36.
6. Kwak PE, Stasney CR, Hathway J, et al. Knowledge, experience, and anxieties of young classical singers in training. J Voice 2014;28(2):191–5.
7. Salturk Z, Kumral TL, Aydoğdu I, et al. Psychological effects of dysphonia in voice professionals. Laryngoscope 2015;125:1908–10.
8. Davies L, Welch HG. Increasing incidence of thyroid cancer in the United States, 1973-2002. JAMA 2016;295:2164–7.
9. Marawar S, Girardi FP, Sama AA, et al. National trends in anterior cervical fusion procedures. Spine (Phila Pa 1976) 2010;35:1454–9.
10. Verdolini K, Ramig LO. Review: occupational risks for voice problems. Logoped Phoniatr Vocol 2001;26:37–46.
11. Cohen SM, Kim J, Roy N, et al. Change in diagnosis and treatment following specialty voice evaluation: a national database analysis. Laryngoscope 2015;125:1660–6.
12. Fritz MA, Persky MJ, Fang Y, et al. The accuracy of the laryngopharyngeal reflux diagnosis: utility of the stroboscopic exam. Otolaryngol Head Neck Surg 2016;155:629–34.
13. Keesecker SE, Murry T, Sulica L. Patterns in the evaluation of hoarseness: time to presentation, laryngeal visualization, and diagnostic accuracy. Laryngoscope 2015;125:667–73.
14. Johns MM. Update on the etiology, diagnosis and treatment of vocal fold nodules, polyps and cysts. Curr Opin Otolaryngol Head Neck Surg 2003;11:456–61.
15. Pasquale K, Wiatrak B, Woolley A, et al. Microdebrider versus CO2 laser removal of recurrent respiratory papillomas: a prospective analysis. Laryngoscope 2003;113:139–43.
16. Mattioli F, Menichetti M, Bergamini G, et al. Results of early versus intermediate or delayed voice therapy in patients with unilateral vocal fold paralysis: our experience in 171 patients. J Voice 2015;29(4):455–8.
17. Kiagiadaki D, Remacle M, Lawson G, et al. The effect of voice rest on the outcome of phonosurgery for benign laryngeal lesions: preliminary results of a prospective randomized study. Ann Otol Rhinol Laryngol 2015;124(5):407–12.
18. Johshi A, Johns MM 3rd. Current practices for voice rest recommendations after phonomicrosurgery. Laryngoscope 2018;128(5):1170–5.
19. Clavé P, Terré R, de Kraa M, et al. Approaching oropharyngeal dysphagia. Rev Esp Enferm Dig 2004;96(2):119–31.

20. Humbert IA, Michou E, MacRae PR, et al. Electrical stimulation and swallowing: how much do we know? Semin Speech Lang 2012;33(3):203–16.
21. Langmore SE, Terpenning MS, Schork A, et al. Predictors of aspiration pneumonia: how important is dysphagia? Dysphagia 1998;13(2):69–81.
22. Delegge MH. Aspiration incidence, mortality, and at-risk populations. J Parenter Enteral Nutr 2002;26(6):19–25.
23. Smith CH, Logemann JA, Colangelo LA, et al. Incidence and patient characteristics associ- ated with silent aspiration in the acute care setting. Dysphagia 1999; 14:1–7.
24. Leder SB, Suiter DM, Murray J, et al. Can an oral mechanism examination contribute to the assessment of odds of aspiration? Dysphagia 2013;28(3):370–4.
25. Martin-Harris B, Logemann JA, McMahon S, et al. Clinical utility of the modified barium swallow. Dysphagia 2000;15(3):136–41.
26. Cichero JAY, Lam P, Steele CM, et al. Development of international terminology and definitions for texture-modified foods and thickened fluids used in dysphagia management: the IDDSI framework. Dysphagia 2017;32(2):293–314.
27. Logemann JA. Evaluation and treatment of swallowing disorders. College-Hill Press, San Diego, California, 1983.
28. Speyer R, Baijens L, Heijnen M, et al. Effects of therapy in oropharyngeal dysphagia by speech and language therapists: a systematic review. Dysphagia 2010;25(1):40–65.
29. Burkhead LM, Sapienza CM, Rosenbek JC. Strength-training exercise in dysphagia rehabilitation: Principles, procedures, and directions for future research. Dysphagia 2007;22(3):251–65.
30. Powers WJ, Rabinstein AA, Ackerson T, et al, American Heart Association Stroke Council, on behalf of the A. H. A. S. 2018 guidelines for the early management of patients with acute ischemic stroke: a guideline for healthcare professionals from the American Heart Association/American Stroke Association. Stroke 2018;49(3): e46–110.
31. Mann G, Hankey GJ, Cameron D. Swallowing function after stroke: prognosis and prognostic factors at 6 months. Stroke 1999;30(4):744–8.
32. Douiri A, McKevitt C, Emmett ES, et al. Long-term effects of secondary prevention on cognitive function in stroke patients. Circulation 2013;128(12):1341–8.
33. Cicerone KD, Langenbahn DM, Braden C, et al. Evidence-based cognitive rehabilitation: updated review of the literature from 2003 through 2008. Arch Phys Med Rehabil 2011;92(4):519–30.
34. Ambrose N, Yairi E. Normative disfluency data for early childhood stuttering. J Speech Lang Hear Res 1999;42:895–909.
35. Riley GD. A stuttering severity instrument for children and adults. J Speech Hear Disord 1972;37(3):314–22.
36. Lundgren K, Helm-Estabrooks N, Klein R. Stuttering following acquired brain damage: a review of the literature. J Neurolinguist 2010;23(5):447–54.
37. Brady JP. Drug-induced stuttering: a review of the literature. J Clin Psychopharmacol 1998;18(1):50–4.
38. Theys C, van Wieringen A, Sunaert S, et al. A one year prospective study of neurogenic stuttering following stroke: Incidence and co-occurring disorders. J Commun Disord 2011;44(6):678–87.
39. Finn P, Felsenfeld S. Recovery from stuttering: the contributions of the qualitative research approach. Int J Speech Lang Pathol 2004;6(3):159–66.

40. Metz DE, Schiavetti N, Sacco PR. Acoustic and psychophysical dimensions of the perceived speech naturalness of nonstutterers and posttreatment stutterers. J Speech Hearing Disord 1990;55(3):516–25.

41. O'Brian S, Onslow M, Cream A, et al. The Camperdown Program: Outcomes of a new prolonged-speech treatment model. J Speech, Lang Hear Res 2003;46(4): 933–46.

42. Blomgren M, Roy N, Callister T, et al. Intensive stuttering modification therapy. J Speech Lang Hearing Res 2005;48(3):509.

43. Irani F, Gabel R, Daniels D, et al. The long term effectiveness of intensive stuttering therapy: a mixed methods study. J Fluency Disord 2012;37(3):164–78.

44. Lincoln M, Packman A, Onslow M, et al. An experimental investigation of the effect of altered auditory feedback on the conversational speech of adults who stutter. J Speech, Lang Hear Res 2010;53(5):1122–31.

45. Yaruss JS, Quesal RW, Reeves L, et al. Speech treatment and support group experiences of people who participate in the National Stuttering Association. J Fluency Disord 2002;27(2):115–34.

# Facial Nerve Paralysis

James A. Owusu, MD[a], C. Matthew Stewart, MD, PhD[b],
Kofi Boahene, MD[b],*

### KEYWORDS

- Facial paralysis • Bell palsy • Ramsay hunt • Facial reanimation

### KEY POINTS

- Timely diagnosis and treatment are keys to achieving good outcomes in facial paralysis.
- Facial paralysis that is persistent or progressive requires further evaluation to rule out a neoplasm.
- Corticosteroid therapy should be initiated within 72 hours for suspected Bell palsy and Ramsay Hunt syndrome.
- Facial paralysis can have significant emotional toll on affected patients, leading to social isolation and depression.

## INTRODUCTION

Facial animation is an essential part of human communication and is one of the main means of expressing emotions and providing nonverbal cues. The smile, for example, has been judged as the most important facial expression that reflects positively on both the person smiling and the observer. When the face is paralyzed as a result of a variety of causes, the lost ability to animate the face can be devastating and is often associated with depression, social isolation, and reduced quality of life. Facial expressions in patients with facial paralysis are often perceived as negative by observers even when they are smiling.[1] Compared with normal controls, individuals with facial paralysis are often judged as unattractive.[1] Besides the psychosocial penalties, facial paralysis significantly impairs essential facial functions, including blinking, cornea protection, nasal breathing, lip competence and speech, and smiling.

Facial animation is orchestrated by the facial muscles directed by the facial nucleus through a network of the facial nerve and its branches. Impairment of any of these components of facial animation can result in partial or complete facial paralysis. Establishing the cause of the facial paralysis gives essential information about

Financial Disclosure: None.
Conflicts of Interest: None.
[a] Department of Head and Neck Surgery, Mid-Atlantic Permanente Medical Group, 8008 Westpark Drive, McLean, VA 22102, USA; [b] Department of Otorhinolaryngology–Head and Neck Surgery, Johns Hopkins Hospital, 601 North Caroline Street, Baltimore, MD 21287, USA
* Corresponding author.
*E-mail address:* dboahen1@jhmi.edu

the prognosis and expected course of the paralysis. The causes of facial paralysis vary broadly but can be categorized as a developmental anomaly or acquired injury affecting the facial nerve, facial muscles, or both. Developmental abnormalities can occur in isolation or as part of a syndrome. Early childhood infection or traumatic birth injuries resulting in facial paralysis should be differentiated from true developmental paralysis. Distinguishing between the 2 causes is important because it influences the type of evaluation and treatment offered. Identifying developmental facial paralysis allows early targeted screening, accurate diagnosis, and prompt referral for treatment in this population, which will facilitate their emotional and social rehabilitation and reintegration among their peers. An example of a development cause of facial paralysis is Möbius syndrome, which has an incidence of 1 per 50,000 births.[2] Another common developmental facial paralysis is the congenital unilateral lower lip palsy, also known as neonatal asymmetric crying facies that occurs in 1 out of 160 live births.[3]

Acquired causes of facial paralysis include vascular compression of the facial nerve, ischemic injuries to the facial motor centers, inflammatory and degenerative processes, primary and secondary neoplasms of the facial nerve, iatrogenic facial nerve injuries, and trauma. Interruption of the neuromuscular pathway from the facial motor cortex to the facial muscles is the finding common to the various causes of facial paralysis. The level at which the pathologic interruption occurs and the resulting functional deficit determines the treatment offered. Restoring facial tone and animation of the paralyzed face requires restoration of the interrupted nerve muscle network by either spontaneous regeneration of the facial nerves or surgical repair of the impaired nerves or muscles.

## CAUSES OF FACIAL PARALYSIS

The causes of facial paralysis vary widely, but can be categorized into the following:

- Idiopathic facial paralysis (Bell palsy [BP], Ramsay Hunt syndrome [RHS])
- Infectious (Lyme disease, otitis media)
- Paralysis resulting from tumors (facial neuroma, acoustic neuroma, geniculate hemangioma, parotid neoplasms)
- Developmental (Mobius, hemi facial microsomia)
- Traumatic (forceps delivery, temporal bone fracture, penetrating injuries: dog bite, stab wound, gunshot injuries)
- Iatrogenic (postsurgical)

## EVALUATING THE PARALYZED FACE

Evaluation of the facial paralysis patient begins with a comprehensive history and physical examination to determine the cause, extent, and duration of paralysis and functional impairment present. History should determine the onset, progression, associated symptoms, and risk factors. A comprehensive examination of the head and neck, including an assessment of all branches of the facial nerve and other cranial nerves, palpation of the parotid gland and the neck, should be performed. Observing the face in repose and in voluntary motion assesses the degree of paralysis. The patient is asked to elevate eyebrow, close eyes, frown, and smile, pucker the lips, puff cheeks, and tense the neck to assess the platysma. The face is observed for synkinesis, which is an indication of aberrant nerve regeneration. The external ear is examined for the presence of vesicles or rashes, which may indicate RHS. The degree of facial paralysis can be graded using standard grading scales, such as the House Brackmann scale.[4] Photographs and videos of the face are very important in documenting the facial function at presentation and progression before and after treatment. Images and videos should capture brow elevation, blink efficiency, eyelid closure, facial tone at rest, and upper and lower lip movement with animation.

A thorough history is usually adequate to determine the cause of facial paralysis. When necessary, a high-resolution MRI or computed tomographic scan may be obtained to evaluate the intracranial and extracranial course of the facial nerve and to evaluate for skeletal and soft tissue abnormalities. Even after a thorough history and high-resolution imaging studies, the cause of a facial paralysis may remain elusive, and a diagnostic surgical exploration may be necessary to rule out occult neoplasms.[5] Occult neoplasms masquerading as BP commonly result in delayed diagnosis and treatment, with the patient presenting with advanced disease that is often incurable. Facial paralysis that is not acute in timing but sequentially affects adjacent facial nerve branches is usually not BP. Paralysis limited to the lower facial muscles with intact forehead animation is usually a sign of a central lesion. Because of bilateral innervation of the forehead muscles, a central lesion spares the forehead muscles. Forehead sparing can also result from a peripheral lesion that involves only the lower division of the facial nerve. A further distinguishing finding is preservation of emotional facial motion with central facial paralysis, whereas peripheral facial paralysis impairs both voluntary and emotional facial animation.[6]

## ELECTRODIAGNOSTIC TESTING

Electrophysiologic studies are helpful in determining the functional status of the facial nerve and muscles. Electroneurography (ENoG) is useful in the setting of unilateral facial paralysis. ENoG involves electrical stimulation of the facial nerve at the stylomastoid foramen and measuring the motor response at the nasolabial fold. The response obtained from stimulating the normal side is compared with that of the paralyzed side. Greater than 90% degeneration on the paralyzed side is associated with a poor chance of recovery. ENoG is performed after 72 hours following nerve injury to allow time for Wallerian degeneration. ENoG is useful in the early phase of acute onset facial paralysis. In long-standing facial paralysis, electromyography (EMG) is a more useful study. EMG detects facial muscle activity using surface or needle electrodes to record motor unit action potentials. Fibrillation potentials are the action potentials of a single muscle fiber that occur spontaneously or after movement of a needle electrode within the muscle fiber. Fibrillation potentials fire at a constant rate, and their presence indicates muscle motor unit denervation. The amplitude of fibrillation waveforms can also give an indication of the duration of denervation. The amplitude of fibrillation potentials drops the longer the muscle is denervated. As a rule, large-fibrillation amplitudes suggest recent injury, and small amplitude indicates injury 6 months or longer. Normal motor units have diphasic or triphasic waveforms. One of the earliest signs of muscle reinnervation is the increase in phases of motor unit recordings. Polyphasic potentials are abnormal action potential waveforms showing 5 or more phases and suggest motor unit reinnervation. Electrical silence is observed in completely denervated muscles, with fibrosis indicating a nonfunctional motor end plate.[7]

In general, although these electrophysiologic studies provide some prognostic information about the status of the facial nerves and facial muscle, they rarely alter the treatment needed for restoring satisfactory movement to the paralyzed face. They should therefore not delay referral to a specialist for prompt intervention.

## COMMON CAUSES OF FACIAL PARALYSIS
### Idiopathic (Bell Palsy)

BP is the most common cause of acute unilateral facial nerve paralysis. It is considered to be idiopathic, although reactivation of latent herpes virus infection in the geniculate ganglion is the leading suspected cause of BP.[8] Viral infection results in inflammation and edema of the facial nerve. Swelling of the facial nerve within the rigid bony fallopian canal results in vascular compromise of the nerve particularly along the labyrinthine segment. The vascular compromise results in degeneration of the facial nerve and secondary changes in the facial nucleus. BP presents acutely and progresses over the course of 3 to 7 days. Although typically self-limited, the facial paresis/paralysis that occurs in BP may cause significant temporary oral incompetence and an inability to close the eyelid, leading to potential eye injury.

In 2013, the American Academy of Otolaryngology-Head and Neck Surgery Foundation published clinical practice guidelines aimed to improve the quality of care and outcomes for patients diagnosed with BP.[9]

The guidelines made a strong recommendation that clinicians (a) should assess the patient using history and physical examination to exclude identifiable causes of facial paresis or paralysis in patients presenting with acute-onset unilateral facial paresis or paralysis, (b) should prescribe oral steroids within 72 hours of symptom onset for patients older than 16 years, (c) should not prescribe oral antiviral therapy alone but only in combination with oral steroids, if at all offered, and (d) should implement eye protection for BP patients with impaired eye closure. The panel recommended (a) against routine laboratory testing, (b) against routine diagnostic imaging, and (c) that clinicians should not perform electrodiagnostic testing in BP patients with incomplete facial paralysis.

Several studies have shown that the status of facial nerve function reflected by the grade, number, and severity of associated symptoms during the first month most accurately predicts extent of recovery at 6 to 12 months in BP.[10]

### Infectious

Herpes zoster oticus and Lyme disease are the most common infectious causes of facial paralysis. Other less common causes include human immunodeficiency virus and otitis media. Herpes zoster oticus arises from reactivation of latent varicella-zoster virus in the geniculate ganglion. It presents as acute facial paralysis with associated otalgia, sensorineural hearing loss, vertigo, and vesicular eruptions of the external ear. Facial paralysis with vesicular eruptions of the ear is known as RHS. RHS has a more protracted course compared with BP, and symptoms can worsen over several weeks. RHS is treated with antivirals such as valacyclovir, famciclovir, and acyclovir combined with steroids. To be most efficacious, treatment needs to be initiated within 72 hours of onset of symptoms.[11]

Infections of the middle ear and external auditory canal and mastoid can result in facial nerve paralysis. The facial nerve traverses the fallopian canal to exit the stylomastoid foramen. This course places the nerve in close proximity to infectious processes of the temporal bone. Inflammation and edema of the nerve in response to infection compromise the vasculature of the nerve because of the rigid fallopian canal, resulting in facial nerve paralysis. Facial nerve paralysis can be seen in the setting of acute and chronic otitis media, mastoiditis, and malignant otitis externa.[12] In the era of antibiotics, a bacterial cause of facial paralysis is rare and mostly limited to neglected cases.

Lyme disease is a multisystemic tick-borne disease caused by the spirochete Borrelia burgdorferi. Facial paralysis can be seen in up to 11% of patients with Lyme disease. Lyme disease should be considered in children presenting with facial paralysis as well as in cases of bilateral facial palsy. Lyme disease is diagnosed with serologic testing and treated with antibiotics. There is good prognosis for full recovery for the patient diagnosed and treated in the early phase of the disease.[12,13]

### Neoplastic

Tumors of the facial nerves and its surrounding structures can compromise the function of the nerve, resulting in facial nerve paralysis. Tumor-related facial paralysis may be classified as primary or secondary. Primary tumors of the facial nerve are fairly rare. The most common primary facial nerve tumors are benign neuromas and hemangiomas. Malignant tumors from the facial skin, parotid gland, and surrounding structure can directly infiltrate or compress the facial nerve, resulting in paresis or paralysis. Metastatic breast, lung, and renal cancer have been known to cause facial paralysis. Benign tumors that commonly affect facial nerves include benign tumors of the parotid gland, glomus tumors, meningiomas, and acoustic neuroma. Acoustic neuroma is the most frequent tumor in this category.[14–17]

### Trauma

The course of the facial nerve from the brainstem through the temporal bone to the facial muscles places it at risk for traumatic injuries. Facial nerve trauma may result from an accidental source or may be iatrogenic. The extent of paralysis is dependent on the location and degree of injury. Sunderland classification grades nerve injuries on a 5-point scale based on the degree of neural tissue damage. The degree of injury predicts the prognosis. Grade I nerve injury, known as neuropraxia, is a temporary blockage of transmission of nerve signals due to compression or traction on the nerve. Grade I injuries have good prognosis for recovery of normal nerve function. Grade V injuries are complete transection of the nerve and are associated with a poor prognosis.[18] Iatrogenic facial nerve injuries are more common than accidental injuries. Temporal bone fractures account for most accidental injuries. When assessing traumatic facial nerve paralysis, the onset of paralysis is a key determinant of prognosis. Delayed onset paralysis in general has a good prognosis because it indicates an intact nerve with secondary compromise of nerve function due to edema. In contrast, paralysis occurring immediately after trauma portends a higher grade nerve injury with poorer prognosis.

## TREATMENT

Facial paralysis may have a significant emotional toll on patients and can lead to depression. Patients with facial paralysis should be assessed for depression and treated appropriately. The principal tenet that should guide treatment of facial paralysis patients is early diagnosis and early treatment. The delay in treatment is perhaps the single most important factor that affects the long-term outcome of patients with facial paralysis.

There are nonsurgical and surgical options for treating facial paralysis. These treatment modalities are targeted to the entire facial nerve to aid recovery, minimize sequelae, and improve facial form and function.

### Nonsurgical Treatment of Facial Paralysis

As previously noted, patients presenting with acute onset facial paralysis considered to be either BP or RHS should be treated with oral steroids within 72 hours. Antivirals may be added to the course of steroid treatment but should not be used as monotherapy.

Paralysis of the eyelid is associated with significant blink inefficiency that can lead to dry eye symptoms with keratitis, corneal abrasion, and possible progression to loss of vision. Corneal protection should be a primary focus of all clinicians managing patients with facial paralysis. Patients should be started on a regimen of topical lubricating drops and ointment. In addition, use of a moisture chamber or eyelid taping may be beneficial in protecting the eye during sleep. Patients with poor cornea sensation fair poorly and often require more aggressive protective measures. There are now available patient-specific cornea-protective shields that are effective in recalcitrant cases. An example is the Prosthetic Replacement of the Ocular Surface Ecosystem.

Patients with facial paralysis often inquire about the role of physical therapy (neuromuscular retraining) to aid their recovery. By itself, physical therapy for the face may not aid the early regeneration of the injured facial nerve but may help in addressing the aberrant regeneration that is commonly associated with severe facial nerve injury. Clinically, aberrant facial nerve regeneration manifests as synkinesis and hyperactivity of the facial muscles. Neuromuscular retraining unlinks undesired motions from desired ones. Because the undesired activity is suppressed, the range of the primary movement gradually extends, increasing excursion, strength, and motor control. Surface EMG, mirror, and video biofeedback help bring desired movements to conscious control. Although there is a paucity of well-designed randomized controlled trials on the effectiveness of facial exercises on the functional outcome of facial paralysis, selected publications support its beneficial role. A systematic review of 132 studies by Pereira and colleagues[19] investigating the role of facial exercises in facial paralysis concluded that it was effective.

Once the patients have become comfortable with self-directed facial retraining exercises, selective chemodenervation with botulinum toxin injection can be beneficial to patients with hemi-facial spasms, synkinesis, or facial muscle hypercontraction.

Facial paralysis patients often complain of difficulties with speech as well and lip competence. They often have bolus spillage when eating or drinking from the paralyzed corner of the mouth. Temporary improvement in this oral phase dysphagia may be achieved with target injection of hyaluronic acid–based filler material into the adynamic lip segment.[20]

### Surgical Treatment of Facial Paralysis

The decision to intervene surgically in patients with facial paralysis is reserved for those patients who are unlikely to make a satisfactory spontaneous recovery after a period of observation or following medical treatment. The timing for surgical intervention is not always clear but should not be delayed. When facial paralysis is a result of a completely disrupted nerve (trauma, surgery), immediate nerve repair is clearly indicated. In cases of facial paralysis when the nerve is anatomically intact (eg, BP, after acoustic neuroma resection with preserved facial nerve, facial nerve schwannoma, facial nerve hemangioma), it is often hoped that the nerves will spontaneously recover, and a period of observation is recommended. How long this period of observation should be is not clear. Retrospective and prospective studies have shown that patients with anatomically intact facial nerves who show no improvement after 6 months of observation are unlikely to make satisfactory long-term recovery and should be considered for reanimation surgery.[21]

### Facial Reanimation

Several reanimation techniques are available and can be broadly classified as static or dynamic. Static procedures suspend the soft tissue structures of the paralyzed face to improve symmetry without providing active motion. Dynamic procedures restore animation to the face using innervated muscles. Dynamic procedures include primary facial nerve repair, nerve grafting, nerve transposition, MTU transposition, and free functional neuromuscular unit transfer. A combination of static and dynamic procedures is usually required to restore facial balance and function. The technique selected for restoring animation to the paralyzed face depends on the functional status of the facial muscles, the health of the patient, and their acceptance of the risks, benefits, and complexity of repair techniques. In general, patients with facial muscles that are physiologically viable benefit from nerve grafting procedures to reestablish innervation of the paralyzed muscle. When the facial muscles are denervated for too long, atrophic, fibrotic, or developmentally abnormal, dynamic facial movement can only be restored with a functional muscle transfer procedure.

### Nerve Grafting Techniques

In general, nerve grafts reestablish neural continuity between the paralyzed facial muscle and the facial motor nucleus. When feasible, the paralyzed facial muscle should be reconnected with the ipsilateral facial nucleus either by direct nerve repair or with a nerve graft. When the ipsilateral facial nucleus cannot be surgically recruited or is functionally unavailable, alternate donor nerves are considered. Commonly recruited donor cranial nerves include the contralateral facial nerve via a cross-facial nerve graft, the masseter nerve, and the hypoglossal nerve.

### Functional Muscle Transfer

When the facial muscles are irreversibly injured or congenitally absent, transfer of functional muscle units is necessary to restore or establish facial animation. Functional muscle units can be transferred as a pedicled muscle tendon unit (MTU) or as a free functional muscle flap (FFMF) that requires microsurgical revascularization and nerve anastomosis. In MTU transfer, the tendon of a functioning muscle is detached, mobilized, and reinserted into another tendon or bone to substitute for the action of a nonfunctioning muscle. The motor nerve and blood supply of the transferred MTU remain intact. The temporalis muscle is commonly transferred as an MTU to restore upper lip symmetry and motion. In this procedure, the temporalis tendon is detached from the coronoid process of the mandible and transposed through the buccal space to suspend the oral commissure and lip. Movement of the temporalis muscle now produces movement of the lip for smiling and tone for midfacial support. Temporalis MTU transfer is an effective means of restoring symmetry, tone, and movement to the midface.

Compared with pedicled MTU, FFMFs are more versatile. The gracilis flap is the most common FFMF used in contemporary facial reanimation surgery for smile restoration. As a substitute donor muscle, the gracilis muscle generates adequate force and excursion for facial support and smile restoration. The gracilis muscle flap is harvested as a small muscle flap and transplanted into the paralyzed face, revascularized, and innervated using microsurgical techniques. The gracilis flap is commonly designed as a single paddle with univector excursion often mimicking the outward contraction of the zygomaticus major muscle. Recent advances have led to the harvest and transplant of the gracilis muscle in a multivector fashion to produce a more realistic smile.[22]

### Static Suspension

Static suspension techniques provide support to the ptotic face and can improve facial symmetry at rest but do not provide any dynamic animation. They may be used in isolation or in combination with other dynamic reanimation techniques. Static procedures include brow lift and facial fascia slings.

### Static Eyelid Procedures

Loading the upper eyelid with an implant is a common means of improving or correcting lagophthalmos. Upper eyelid loading is partly recommended for its effect on blink efficiency. Complete and efficient blink distributes protective tear film over the ocular surface, which is essential for corneal health. Upper eyelid loading is more effective when combined with blink efficiency exercises. Patients are encouraged to consciously practice voluntary blinking with a focus on reproducing the attributes of an effective blink: full and complete, relaxed and light, rapid and natural. Gold and platinum eyelid implants are the most commonly used eyelid implants.

### Lower Eyelid Suspension Sling

The retracted lower eyelid can also be vertically suspended with fascia slings placed along the margin of the lower eyelid and anchored medially and laterally. Facial sling may be obtained from the fascia lata or from the deep temporal fascia. The sling is placed deep to the orbicularis oculi muscle and secured to periosteum lateral and superior to the attachment points of the canthal ligaments.

### Intermarginal Adhesion

Tarsorrhaphy is closure of the eyelids via an adhesion between the 2 upper and lower lid margins, which reduces corneal exposure and evaporation of the tear film. It involves creating 2 opposing raw surfaces along the upper and lower eye lid margin. The raw edges are sutured together to create an adhesion. It is technically straightforward and is a reversible procedure.

### Synkinesis

Facial synkinesis is a distressing manifestation of aberrant facial nerve regeneration following facial paralysis. Synkinesis refers to the abnormal, unwanted, involuntary facial movement that occurs coupled with purposeful facial movement. For example, oro-ocular synkinesis occurs when movement of the lips results in closure of the eyelids. Mild forms of synkinesis may go undetected, but severe forms cannot be ignored because they may cause severe facial pain and facial tightness. The treatment of facial synkinesis is one of the most challenging aspects of facial paralysis care. Facial retraining exercises are recommended to help suppress unwanted movement. Selective chemodenervation with botulinum toxin is the most common treatment modality.

### SUMMARY

Facial nerve paralysis can have a significant physical and emotional toll on affected individuals. A thorough history and physical examination are needed to narrow the broad differential diagnosis and determine an appropriate management plan. Timely intervention is needed to provide patients the best chance for recovery of normal nerve function. Eye care should be initiated in all patients with facial nerve paralysis and signs of incomplete eye closure.

### REFERENCES

1. Ishii L, Godoy A, Encarnacion CO, et al. Not just another face in the crowd: society's perceptions of facial paralysis. Laryngoscope 2012;122(3):533–8.

2. Verzijl HT, Van Der Zwaag B, Cruysberg JR, et al. Möbius syndrome redefined: a syndrome of rhombencephalic maldevelopment. Neurology 2003;61(3):327–33.
3. Sapin SO, Miller A, Bass HN. Neonatal asymmetric crying faces: a new look at an old problem. Clin Pediatr 2005;44:109–19.
4. House JW, Brackmann DE. Facial nerve grading system. Otolaryngol Head Neck Surg 1985;93(2):146–7.
5. Boahene DO, Olsen KD, Driscoll C, et al. Facial nerve paralysis secondary to occult malignant neoplasms. Otolaryngol Head Neck Surg 2004;130(4):459–65.
6. Töpper R, Kosinski C, Mull M. Volitional type of facial palsy associated with pontine ischaemia. J Neurol Neurosurg Psychiatry 1995;58:732–4.
7. Valls-Sole J. Electrodiagnostic studies of the facial nerve in a peripheral facial palsy and hemifacial spasm. Muscle Nerve 2007;36(1):14–20.
8. Schirm J, Mulkens PS. Bell's palsy and herpes simplex virus. APMIS 1997;105: 815–23.
9. Baugh RF, Basura GJ, Ishii LE, et al. Clinical practice guideline: Bell's palsy. Otolaryngol Head Neck Surg 2013;149:S1–27.
10. Holland NJ, Weiner GM. Recent developments in Bell's palsy. BMJ 2004; 329(7465):553–7.
11. Robillard RB, Hilsinger RL Jr, Adour KK. Ramsay hunt facial paralysis: clinical analyses of 185 patients. Otolaryngol Head Neck Surg 1986;95:292–7.
12. Makeham TP, Croxson GR, Coulson S. Infective causes of facial nerve paralysis. Otol Neurotol 2007;28(1):100–3.
13. Clark JR, Carlson RD, Sasaki CT, et al. Facial paralysis in Lyme disease. Laryngoscope 1985;95:1341–5.
14. Pillsbury HC, Price HC, Gardiner LJ. Primary tumors of facial nerve. Laryngoscope 1983;93:1045–8.
15. Pulec JL. Facial nerve neuroma. Ear Nose Throat J 1994;73:721–52.
16. Selesnick SH, Burt BM. Regional spread of nonneurogenic tumors to the skull base via the facial nerve. Otol Neurotol 2003;24:326–33.
17. Suryanarayanan R, Dezso A, Ramsden RT, et al. Metastatic carcinoma mimicking a facial nerve schwannoma: the role of computerized tomography in diagnosis. J Laryngol Otol 2005;119:1010–2.
18. Sunderland S. A classification of peripheral nerve injuries producing loss of function. Brain 1951;74(4):491–516.
19. Pereira LM, Obara K, Dias JM, et al. Facial exercise therapy for facial palsy: systematic review and meta-analysis. Clin Rehabil 2011;25:649–58.
20. Starmer H, Lyford-Pike S, Ishii LE, et al. Quantifying labial strength and function in facial paralysis: effect of targeted lip injection augmentation. JAMA Facial Plast Surg 2015;17:274–8.
21. Rivas A, Boahene KD, Bravo HC, et al. A model for early prediction of facial nerve recovery after vestibular schwannoma surgery. Otol Neurotol 2011;32:826–33.
22. Boahene KO, Owusu J, Ishii L, et al. The multivector gracilis free functional muscle flap for facial reanimation. JAMA Facial Plast Surg 2018. https://doi.org/10.1001/jamafacial.2018.0048.

# UNITED STATES POSTAL SERVICE ® Statement of Ownership, Management, and Circulation
## (All Periodicals Publications Except Requester Publications)

| 1. Publication Title | 2. Publication Number | 3. Filing Date |
|---|---|---|
| MEDICAL CLINICS IN NORTH AMERICA | 337 – 340 | 9/18/2018 |

| 4. Issue Frequency | 5. Number of Issues Published Annually | 6. Annual Subscription Price |
|---|---|---|
| JAN, MAR, MAY, JUL, SEP, NOV | 6 | $5273.00 |

7. Complete Mailing Address of Known Office of Publication (Not printer) (Street, city, county, state, and ZIP+4®)

ELSEVIER INC.
230 Park Avenue, Suite 800
New York, NY 10169

Contact Person: STEPHEN R. BUSHING
Telephone (Include area code): 215-239-3688

8. Complete Mailing Address of Headquarters or General Business Office of Publisher (Not printer)

ELSEVIER INC.
230 Park Avenue, Suite 800
New York, NY 10169

9. Full Names and Complete Mailing Addresses of Publisher, Editor, and Managing Editor (Do not leave blank)

Publisher (Name and complete mailing address)

TAYLOR E. BALL, ELSEVIER INC.
1600 JOHN F KENNEDY BLVD. SUITE 1800
PHILADELPHIA, PA 19103-2899

Editor (Name and complete mailing address)

JESSICA MCCOOL, ELSEVIER INC.
1600 JOHN F KENNEDY BLVD. SUITE 1800
PHILADELPHIA, PA 19103-2899

Managing Editor (Name and complete mailing address)

PATRICK MANLEY, ELSEVIER INC.
1600 JOHN F KENNEDY BLVD. SUITE 1800
PHILADELPHIA, PA 19103-2899

10. Owner (Do not leave blank. If the publication is owned by a corporation, give the name and address of the corporation immediately followed by the names and addresses of all stockholders owning or holding 1 percent or more of the total amount of stock. If not owned by a corporation, give the names and addresses of the individual owners. If owned by a partnership or other unincorporated firm, give its name and address as well as those of each individual owner. If the publication is published by a nonprofit organization, give its name and address.)

| Full Name | Complete Mailing Address |
|---|---|
| WHOLLY OWNED SUBSIDIARY OF REED/ELSEVIER, US HOLDINGS | 1600 JOHN F KENNEDY BLVD. SUITE 1800 PHILADELPHIA, PA 19103-2899 |

11. Known Bondholders, Mortgagees, and Other Security Holders Owning or Holding 1 Percent or More of Total Amount of Bonds, Mortgages, or Other Securities. If none, check box ▶ ☐ None

| Full Name | Complete Mailing Address |
|---|---|
| N/A | |

12. Tax Status (For completion by nonprofit organizations authorized to mail at nonprofit rates) (Check one)
The purpose, function, and nonprofit status of this organization and the exempt status for federal income tax purposes:
☒ Has Not Changed During Preceding 12 Months
☐ Has Changed During Preceding 12 Months (Publisher must submit explanation of change with this statement)

PS Form 3526, July 2014 (Page 1 of 4 (see instructions page 4)) PSN: 7530-01-000-9931 PRIVACY NOTICE: See our privacy policy on www.usps.com.

---

| 13. Publication Title | 14. Issue Date for Circulation Data Below |
|---|---|
| MEDICAL CLINICS IN NORTH AMERICA | JULY 2018 |

| 15. Extent and Nature of Circulation | | | Average No. Copies Each Issue During Preceding 12 Months | No. Copies of Single Issue Published Nearest to Filing Date |
|---|---|---|---|---|
| a. Total Number of Copies (Net press run) | | | 487 | 685 |
| b. Paid Circulation (By Mail and Outside the Mail) | (1) | Mailed Outside-County Paid Subscriptions Stated on PS Form 3541 (Include paid distribution above nominal rate, advertiser's proof copies, and exchange copies) | 263 | 330 |
| | (2) | Mailed In-County Paid Subscriptions Stated on PS Form 3541 (Include paid distribution above nominal rate, advertiser's proof copies, and exchange copies) | 0 | 0 |
| | (3) | Paid Distribution Outside the Mails Including Sales Through Dealers and Carriers, Street Vendors, Counter Sales, and Other Paid Distribution Outside USPS® | 126 | 223 |
| | (4) | Paid Distribution by Other Classes of Mail Through the USPS (e.g., First-Class Mail®) | 0 | 0 |
| c. Total Paid Distribution [Sum of 15b (1), (2), (3), and (4)] | | ▶ | 391 | 553 |
| d. Free or Nominal Rate Distribution (By Mail and Outside the Mail) | (1) | Free or Nominal Rate Outside-County Copies Included on PS Form 3541 | 83 | 114 |
| | (2) | Free or Nominal Rate In-County Copies Included on PS Form 3541 | 0 | 0 |
| | (3) | Free or Nominal Rate Copies Mailed at Other Classes Through the USPS (e.g., First-Class Mail) | 0 | 0 |
| | (4) | Free or Nominal Rate Distribution Outside the Mail (Carriers or other means) | 0 | 0 |
| e. Total Free or Nominal Rate Distribution (Sum of 15d (1), (2), (3) and (4)) | | ▶ | 83 | 114 |
| f. Total Distribution (Sum of 15c and 15e) | | ▶ | 474 | 667 |
| g. Copies not Distributed (See Instructions to Publishers #4 (page #3)) | | ▶ | 13 | 18 |
| h. Total (Sum of 15f and g) | | | 487 | 685 |
| i. Percent Paid (15c divided by 15f times 100) | | | 82.49% | 82.91% |

* If you are claiming electronic copies, go to line 16 on page 3. If you are not claiming electronic copies, skip to line 17 on page 3.

| 16. Electronic Copy Circulation | | Average No. Copies Each Issue During Preceding 12 Months | No. Copies of Single Issue Published Nearest to Filing Date |
|---|---|---|---|
| a. Paid Electronic Copies | ▶ | 0 | 0 |
| b. Total Paid Print Copies (Line 15c) + Paid Electronic Copies (Line 16a) | ▶ | 391 | 553 |
| c. Total Print Distribution (Line 15f) + Paid Electronic Copies (Line 16a) | ▶ | 474 | 667 |
| d. Percent Paid (Both Print & Electronic Copies) (16b divided by 16c × 100) | ▶ | 82.49% | 82.91% |

☒ I certify that 50% of all my distributed copies (electronic and print) are paid above a nominal price.

17. Publication of Statement of Ownership

☒ If the publication is a general publication, publication of this statement is required. Will be printed in the NOVEMBER 2018 issue of this publication. ☐ Publication not required.

| 18. Signature and Title of Editor, Publisher, Business Manager, or Owner | | Date |
|---|---|---|
| Stephen R. Bushing — Stephen R. Bushing - Inventory Distribution Control Manager | | 9/18/2018 |

I certify that all information furnished on this form is true and complete. I understand that anyone who furnishes false or misleading information on this form or who omits material or information requested on the form may be subject to criminal sanctions (including fines and imprisonment) and/or civil sanctions (including civil penalties).

PS Form 3526, July 2014 (Page 3 of 4) PRIVACY NOTICE: See our privacy policy on www.usps.com.

# Moving?

## Make sure your subscription moves with you!

To notify us of your new address, find your **Clinics Account Number** (located on your mailing label above your name), and contact customer service at:

**Email: journalscustomerservice-usa@elsevier.com**

**800-654-2452** (subscribers in the U.S. & Canada)
**314-447-8871** (subscribers outside of the U.S. & Canada)

**Fax number: 314-447-8029**

**Elsevier Health Sciences Division**
**Subscription Customer Service**
**3251 Riverport Lane**
**Maryland Heights, MO 63043**

*To ensure uninterrupted delivery of your subscription, please notify us at least 4 weeks in advance of move.